Shaken Not Stirred...

A Chemo Cocktail

by Joules Evans

(A Comedy About My Tragedy)

Printed in the United States of America

ISBN: 978-1466452794 (paperback)

This title will also be made available in audiobook, eBook, and hardback editions. For more information, or to contact the author: www.joulesevans.com

Acknowledgments (soundtrack credits) for Shaken Not Stirred…A Chemo Cocktail Mix appear beginning on page 236 I'm a fan of all the music now playing in this Chemo Cocktail Mix of a book and have done my best to honor the artists and their intellectual property by giving them both credit and kudos. Please help me pay forward my gratitude by downloading the iTunes mix.

Apologies: I'm not a doctor and as such am not trying to dispense medical advice. So please take my medical experience with two grains of sea salt and don't call me too early in the morning.
I'm not a perfect Christ follower, nor do I even claim to be a good one, so if I've caused offense in any way, by my irreverent reverence (or vice versa), that is the *last* thing I meant to do. I beg your forgiveness and that you not hold anything I've said or done against the one I follow with all my heart despite my stumbling steps.

Cover Design: Mikeyy Evans: mike@evanshire.net
Cover Cartoon Art: London Glover: grsanatomy09@aol.com
Cover Photography: Jennie Beard: www.jbfreshphotography.com

To Dave.

What in the world would I have done if I hadn't said "I do"?
Sorry I cashed "in sickness" chips.
Hope things are "for better" now.

To Amanda, Matt, and Mikeyy.

You are my three reasons.
Sorry to be such a drama queen of a mum with all this cancer crap, not to mention, the Vespa incident. You may feel like nobody noticed everything you went through while your mum had cancer, but for what it's worth, I totally noticed. Everything. And I'm so sorry you had to go through so much. Too much. But know that you have risen up and blessed me. Never has a mum had such tlc.

Let's go to Chow Fun, K?

"Though the mountains be shaken
and the hills be removed,
yet my unfailing love for you will not be shaken
nor my covenant of peace be removed,"
says the LORD*, who has compassion on you.*

Isaiah 54:10

TABLE OF CONTENTS
(THE PLAYLIST[1])

PART I – SHAKEN NOT STIRRED

PART II – A CHEMO COCKTAIL

PART III – HANGOVER

---

[1] Soundtrack credits begin on page 236.

Part I – Shaken Not Stirred

Chapter 1
Born to Laugh

When I was a kid, I wanted to be a CIA agent when I grew up. I invented a spy persona and called myself Joules Bond, 006.910111213.[2]

Here are a few declassified photos from my dossier. Clearly I took my bottles shaken not stirred and my knack for assuming secret identities was also apparently pre-programmed.

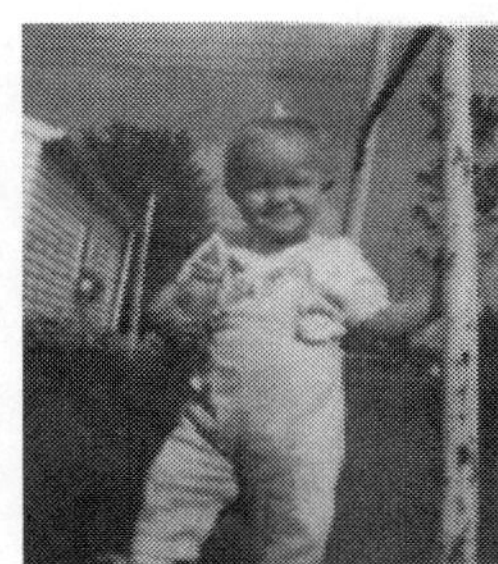
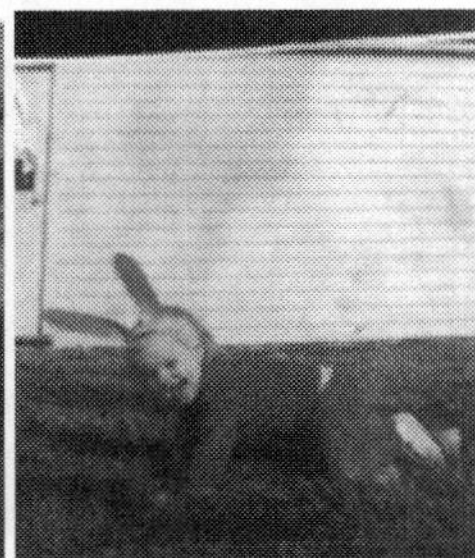
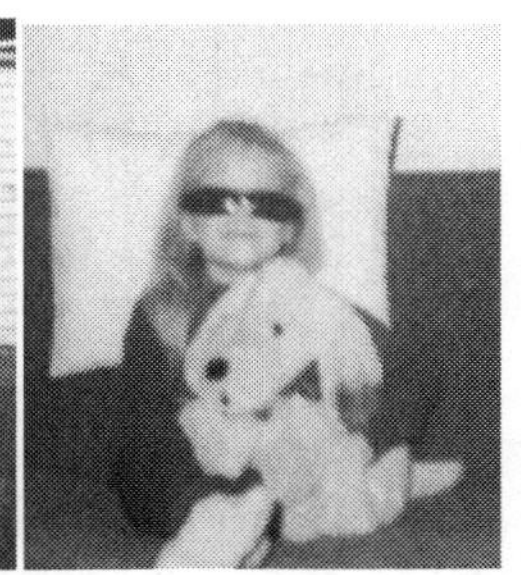

Even from the womb, it seems I had an alias way before I ever had a real name—in utero I went by Jeffrey Scott because my parents thought they were having a boy.

Boy, was I a surprise!

I don't know if you saw the pilot episode of *Alias* or not, but for me, watching it felt like déjà vu.

I wouldn't have blinked an eye, if a couple of men in dark suits and sunglasses had nonchalantly sauntered into my junior high school cafeteria, plopped their trays down at my table—conveniently bumping my tray and scattering a few French fries—while covertly sliding an apparently blank business card (the old "invisible ink trick" of course) into the palm of my hand. "What's the mystery meat today?" one of them would say, which, of course, would be code for "Check the bottom of your milk carton," which would just have the word *napkin* on it. At which point I would discreetly remove my napkin from the silverware tray and unroll its contents, pretending to need my spoon for the rice pudding. (I really did love that rice pudding.) But this was quite possibly national security at stake, so I would down the pudding STAT! and then, while wiping my mouth, quickly scan the note, which would explain that I fit the perfect profile to be the perfect spy.

Smooth intro. With an embedded P.S. of an urgent plea to join the agency. Followed by encoded instructions that, *should I choose to accept this mission*, I should signify by swallowing the napkin—before it self-destructs in ten seconds and causes a scene in the cafeteria. Then I should call the number on the card at my earliest convenience to set up our next rendezvous, at which point I would be filled in as to the details of my first mission.

My eyes were peeled for those guys to finally show.

I remember the summer that one of my oldest childhood friends, Monica, and I took on the Case of the Missing Link. I had no idea what the missing link was. I hadn't taken biology yet. (Not that it would've mattered. I've never been the scientist type—*always* the spy type.) Anyway, Monica hooked me at the first mention of *the missing link*. It sounded so mysterious, so cool—how could we not take the case? We had trench coats and magnifying glasses and notepads and clue-sniffing hounds. We tracked the case all summer long.

Eventually, though, the yellow buses started coming around again, and they chased away the summer. As the daze faded, so the case grew cold. Also we got interested in boys. And roller skating. And especially roller skating with boys.

Seventh grade was probably my most productive year of spy ops training. I had recruited a friend named Kim. We spent much of our latchkey moments on the phone compiling lists of cool words in pocket-sized notebooks, which we carried around and used like they were secret codes. That following summer, she went to Florida with my family on vacation. We assumed secret identities and accents and stayed in character the entire trip.[3] I think we drove my mother nuts with it all but she didn't really say anything about it. It's entirely possible that the "respectable distance" she kept from us whenever we were in public was in reality embarrassment. At the time, though, I gave her mad props for not blowing our cover.

By eighth grade I was so primed for the spy life that I thought I'd better invest a little more in inventing and substantiating my back-story and parallel life. So I went on "official record" that I wanted to be a clerk for a Supreme Court justice when I grew up. My English teacher was filming our campaigns, I mean, class speeches about what we wanted to be when we grew up, so the opportunity just presented itself. I said it right to the camera. From there my course was set, and I followed through with it, almost to a tee. Practically a double major in college: I ended up with the emphasis on my journalism degree and one course short of a second degree in political science. "Missed it by that much!" as Maxwell Smart would've said.

The G-Men never showed.

Well, it's probably for the best. As much as I would like to think that I could have been a great spy, I know I'm wired like one, and maybe, just maybe, the makers of *Alias* modeled the Sydney Bristow character after me. The truth is, I'm probably a little bit more like Maxwell Smart. "Aaand loving it!" There's something about "that old [comedy] trick" that gets me every single time. I do drama—ask my kids, my Redheads as I call them—but besides driving them crazy, the drama is mostly unintentional—as in, dramatic irony often happens to me. But it usually happens to have an element of comedy in it. Lucky for me, I have an innate love of comedy.

It's like I was born to laugh or something.

I thought I was going to be a super spy when I was a kid. I had no clue I would grow up to have to face such an evil and deadly nemesis: breast cancer. But it was more than drama; it was tragedy. It was a mission (not) impossible, but I am *still* in the process of debriefing. Basically, my postcard from breast cancer says, "Been there, done that . . . had to buy a new T-shirt. Don't wish you were here."

Cancer is a real bitch. The thing is, though, God is really good. The Bible speaks of joy that comes in the morning.[4] I've experienced this deeply in the midst of my cancer.

I was born to laugh and I think God made me this way. I don't know exactly how . . . I think it has to be the grace of God[5] . . . but I have not wallowed in my cancer. I have wailed but not wallowed. I did feel like I was dealing with a lemon when I got the diagnosis. I was definitely shaken. I'm not going to sugarcoat the rim and pretend that cancer was sweet, or anything sick like that. What it *was*, was a twist of my fate I had to figure out how to cope with.

They say when life hands you lemons to make lemonade. Well, I figure when that happens, it's not just five o'clock somewhere, but precisely in the exact spot I'm in. That's why I prefer a lemontini. How's *that* for dramatic irony? The lemon never knows what's coming. And then you throw in the vodka. Now *that's* a twist I can dance.

Shaken, not stirred.

I was born to laugh . . . but . . . I learned to laugh through my tears.[6]

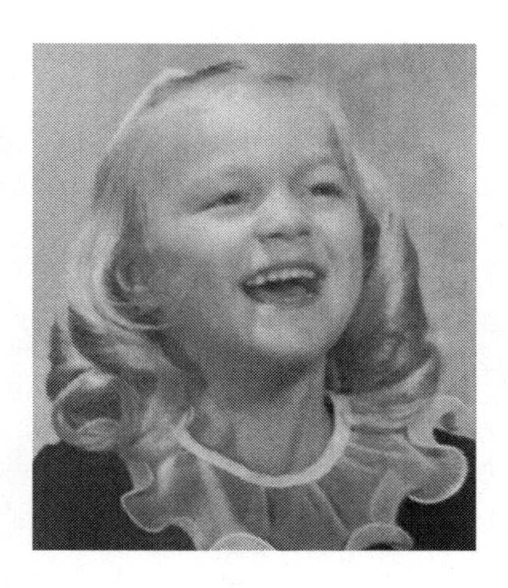

---

[2] Matthew 6:9–13

[3] If you ever saw Steve Martin and Dan Aykroyd play "The Czech Brothers" on Saturday Night Live, well that's why my mum pretended not to know the two wild and crazy girls we were.

[4] Psalm 30:5

[5] 1 Corinthians 15:10

[6] The first and last lines of "Born" by Over the Rhine. If my recording of that song was on vinyl it would be as smooth as my bald head was during chemo. The needle wouldn't be able to find a single groove remaining. That's how many times I listened to it on loop while I was going through cancer.

Chapter 2
When the Stars Go Blue

On August 11, 2008, there were meteor showers over Cincinnati.[7] My world was rocked that night, but it had nothing to do with the meteors that my teenage son Mikeyy and I watched in the wee hours of that sleepless in Cincinnati kind of night.

Previous to Perseus' fireworks display, somewhere in between the lines of August 11 and 12, I'd awakened particularly parched from the end-of-season cocktail party I'd thrown that evening at the *Evanshire,* aka my home sweet home.

Being somewhat of a newbie tennis freak, I'd played on three tennis teams that summer. My neighborhood team had just won the division championship. My United States Tennis Association (USTA) team had just played in the district championship tournament. We actually won the districts, *but.*

And the big but (yeah, they say everybody's got one) was that the win pushed one of our player's ratings into a higher bracket, *which.*

And the "rhymes-with-a-witch" was that "the win?" officially disqualified all her matches and our team from the victory, not to mention a road trip to regionals. The trophy didn't have a chance to slip through our fingers; we never even got to touch it before the ruling came raining down on our parade.

For the cocktail party, I'd grabbed several bottles of a certain Grenache that had caught my eye from across the wine store where I was searching for just the right red and/or white to go with our blues. It had a hot pink label with elegant cursive lettering that read *Bitch*. Bingo! My tennis girlfriends cracked up when I presented the wine. Then we all sighed, and said, "Yeah, it sure was." We uncorked the wine. It was the best of times and we were making the best of the worst of times. We ate and drank and made merry.[8] I went to bed thirsty.

I knew I would wake up in the middle of the night dying-of-thirst thirsty. What I didn't know was that dying of thirst would end up saving my life.

It was five o'clock somewhere—for me it was somewhere in the middle of the night when I woke up from a dream in which I was practically dying of thirst and trying desperately, though unsuccessfully, to quench it.

"Need . . . H . . . 2 . . . Ohhhh," I sputtered out in a dry whisper like I was some kind of a tumbleweed, searching for an oasis.

"So. [click] Very. [click] Thirsty."

I couldn't even peel my tongue off the roof of my mouth.

I'd dealt with similar middle-of-the-night dehydration before, so I had the drill down, practically in my sleep. I tumbled out of bed, crawled across the bedroom floor, slithered down the stairs more like a Slinky than a snake, and somehow found myself standing in front of the kitchen sink. I guzzled a glass of water, diluting the dehydration and dousing the dream. Then I poured another, and headed to the study to sip on the second one while checking Facebook. And I played a little *Scramble*, to try and unscramble the fog in my brain.

That's when I bumped up against my desk—*Ouch*. I felt—and heard—an unexpected thud. *Something* had gone bump in the night—and the bump was on me: my left breast, to be more specific. My jaw fell to the floor and my eyebrows formed a question mark as I held my breath, brought my hand to my breast, and felt the lump.

I cannot explain the shock and awe I felt. It was like a meteor to my chest, literally. I remember the lump felt like a shooter marble right beneath the "milky way." I was pretty sure it wasn't there the day before. My hubby, Dave, didn't mention anything about marbles later that night. I'm sorry if that's TMI, but I don't see how we could've missed a meteor like that.

I don't know how long I sat there trying to imagine what in the world the marble could be. I found myself checking and rechecking to see if it was really there. Then I kept checking and rechecking to see if it was *still* there. Part of me thought I was imagining things. But, no, it was *still* there. Part of me *started* imagining things. I felt the meteor again, and then stared out the window.

My fourteen-year-old son Mikeyy was lying out on the driveway, gazing up at the meteor showers in the sky. I let go of my own gravity and let myself get pulled into his world for a little while—snuggling up next to him and watching the sky fall, like it was a movie.

That time with Mikeyy is etched in my soul as a perfect snapshot of—not my life passing before my eyes, in the dying sense—but more like a haiku, capturing what it was all about.

When the meteor show was over, I had a hard time keeping my thoughts from spiraling out of control. A sensible part of me, that I had to dig way down deep for, took all the other parts of me, and put them to bed.

Not wanting to wake Dave, I lay there, deciding to wait out the night. I waited for him to wake. I waited to see if it would just go away. I waited. And prayed.

Since my thoughts like to play connect the dots, this is where my inner Lady Macbeth spoke up: "Out, damn'd spot" were the words that came out. This seemed like a reasonable prayer, so I went with it.

I spent a lot of time trying to figure out what to say to Dave when he awoke. The truth is, I generally obsess over just about anything I even think of, processing it from every angle before it gets "on deck," on the tip of my tongue. Just to make sure I *say what I mean to say*, and that I *articulate it the way I mean it.* Extroverting is not my strong suit. I can do it, but I don't think I do it very well. And it wears me out. I had nothing by the time he woke up. I was worn out, wound up, and ended up just winging it.

Some words tumbled out into the air and then seemed to settle in a cloud over Dave. He groaned one of those "groanings which cannot be uttered,"[9] (like he already knew, too) and fearfully, mechanically, reached over toward the spot.

Dave said that waking up to that morning was like waking up on the worst possible side of the bed *ever.*

> I was still pretty groggy when Joules asked me about a lump she had found on her breast. She's pretty random and often catches me off guard, but in twenty years of marriage, she had never

> asked anything quite like this. As soon as I felt the obvious lump, the fog instantly cleared and I was wide awake. My heart and mind started racing, but I tried not to let her see my fear. Outside I was saying, "Hmm, that's strange," but inside I was frantically praying, "Please, God, no! Please, God, no! Please, God, no!" Ever since we had a friend diagnosed with breast cancer, I held a secret fear that it might strike Joules one day. This fear only intensified when our friend lost her seven-year battle. Before that, cancer was something other people got. Old people. People with unhealthy lifestyles. People I didn't know. But our friend was young, healthy (fit, even), a wife and mom, a good and godly woman. And she was one of Joules's closest friends. Suddenly breast cancer was very real to me, and very scary.

I won't ever forget that groan. Dave's middle name, Wayne, means *wagon*, and I could just feel him bearing the weight that was to come.

He felt the spot; I had not imagined it.

He got out of bed and made a pot of coffee. Dave makes coffee for me every morning. Even brings a cup up to our bedroom and sets it on my nightstand to help me wake up, smell the coffee, rise and shine, seize the day. Yes, I am spoiled. I admit it.

Then he headed to the study with his computer, and began researching what "not bad" things it could be. At first we were hoping it might be a cyst, or hormones. Or even a boil—at which point, I channeled my inner Job. Then he began adding big words that started with *fibro-* and *pap-* and ended in *-oma*, and my brain went all foggy again.

I poured another cup of coffee and called my sister, Jennie, who lives in Charleston, to tell her about the damn spot. She's my baby sister, but also my best friend. She's also a little ADHD. I happen to love her rabbit trails, so I figured I could thumb a ride on her distraction.

Jennie later described the rabbit hole she fell in when I told her about the lump.

> The day Joules called me and told me about the damn spot she found, I asked her if she thought it might just be a pimple or something weird like that. I tried to be reassuring for her and myself. The thing is, Joules has always been the strong one, and almost like a mother to me, all my life. And to me, nothing bad could or would ever happen to her. But when we hung up the

> phone, the knot that seemed to have tied in my throat came undone, and my tears broke free. My glass is not always as full as my sister's, and it sort of felt like it had just tipped over.

Dave made an appointment with my gynecologist for three o'clock that afternoon. I had chosen her because I was not really into doctors at the time. She was a naturopath, but also an MD. Basically, she was into alternative/non-traditional—with leanings toward Eastern—medicine. I liked that she was not a traditional medical evangelist, but had that training as well, in the palette of her doctor's bag. I did not worry that she would jump to any radical medical conclusions because that was not her holistic style. I felt we were sort of on the same page and that everything *could be* OK, because she was the most likely doctor to find alternative explanations for the spot, and alternative ways of spot removal.

Meanwhile, Dave told me I should go ahead and go to a tennis clinic I'd already signed up and paid for, to try to keep my mind off that damn spot until three.

---

[7] http://science.nasa.gov/science-news/science-at-nasa/2008/22jul_perseiddawn/

[8] Ecclesiastes 8:15

[9] Romans 8:26

Chapter 3
Help Me Out God

I'd never had a mammogram before. *Please* . . . **DO NOT** put it off until you're forty-two years old and find a lump in your breast, like I did.

Dr. Allen couldn't find the spot at first. One would think that would be a good sign. At least, we tried to take it as one. I'm a small-framed person and, to put it frankly, there is not a lot of room for a spot to hide. Maybe my simple prayer had been answered? Maybe I worked the spot out while I played tennis? Or maybe I *had* imagined it, after all.

That would've been awesome. That would've been the end of this story. And there is part of me that would've been OK with that. But that's not how it happened. She eventually found the proverbial *X*.

Damn spot. It had been elusive due to rather awkward placement, right beneath the "milky way." It figures, that even my cells would be undercover—all cloak and dagger, and spies like me.

I could tell that Dr. Allen didn't seem to like what she'd found. She said she thought we should do a mammogram and an ultrasound to "cover second base." That was not what I expected her to say, at all. Then she picked up the phone and scheduled the tests for the very next day.

I wasn't scared yet. I had some adrenaline pumping, but not from jumping to conclusions. The things I'd heard about mammograms, particularly the squashing involved, made me cringe. I'd always experienced a sympathetic twinge of pain whenever I was with a group of women and the conversation uncomfortably shifted to mammogram stories, which usually followed everyone's birth stories.

If you saw *Casino Royale*, you might remember a certain scene in which the most recent James Bond, played by Daniel Craig, took a few torturous knocks to the groin area. I had to close my eyes because I don't like seeing people tortured. Or naked, really. And, especially, not being tortured while naked. The collective gasp from the men in the theater during that scene told me it was one of those need-to-know scenes that I didn't need to know. They obviously felt his pain.

Stories about mammograms and the squashing involved had a similar effect on me. And my overactive imagination did not help things when it came to considering my own impending mammogram. If mammograms were a Facebook page I would not have been a fan. If there were such a thing as a dislike button, I would have pressed it. Yet I needed to know what that damn spot was, so I didn't have the mammogram invite removed from my events.

On Wednesday, my hubby and I went to what is now the Mary Jo Cropper Family Center for Breast Care at Bethesda North Hospital, in Cincinnati, to have the scheduled tests.

I couldn't believe what a big deal my mammogram *wasn't*.[10] In retrospect, it was probably harder on my hubby than it was on me. I mean it. I found myself a tad distracted when the technician took out a Sharpie and drew an *X* right on the spot. Then she remarked that it was at six o'clock on my breast. I have to admit that I did appreciate the poetry of the whole *X* marking the spot. I had an LOL moment, though, when she told me the placement in terms of a clock face. The spot was actually somewhere between 5:27 and 5:28, but I also round up. For some reason, this thought got a hold of my funny bone and wouldn't let go, despite the gravity that kept trying to suck me in. And my funny bone is connected to my coping bone. This is where my head was while I placed my breasts between the mammography plates that squished but did not squash me.

Dave had no distractions and was not finding himself lost in the poetry of the Sharpie's *X*. He was impatiently watching the clock and anxiously pacing off the waiting room like he was Quick Draw

McGraw. Apparently, the nurses got worried about him and asked me to check on him as soon as they finished squishing my breasts between the mammography plates and right before they gelled them up for the ultrasound.

Dave was wound so tight that he had pitted out his shirt. Earlier we'd started a crossword puzzle together, but he couldn't concentrate on it. We decided that it would've been a good thing to stock the waiting room with Scotch—right next to the coffee pot. Dave didn't really need any caffeine. It was only three in the afternoon but we'd already established that it was already almost half-past five o'clock on my breast. Dave could've used a Scotch, maybe a double, and on the double.

The ultrasound was lengthy, due in part to the aforementioned savvy of the spot. But the technician also happened to find two more damn spots, while searching for the *X* that marked the first.

Also, the technician had a bit of a sneezing fit during the process. It was awkward sitting there with freezing cold gel on my hot boobs while the poor girl sneezed her head off. I said "bless you" a few times. The I threw in a "gesundheit." After that I didn't know what to say. So I asked her if she thought she might possibly be allergic to me.

After the tests I remember standing in a very small room while a couple of men in scrubs briefed Dave and me. They said the original spot was about a centimeter, the second was 0.7, and the third was 0.6. They said they all appeared to be solid masses—which didn't sound good. But they tried to reassure us that it was not *necessarily* bad news. They recommended that we biopsy them all, but stressed I should not go home thinking I have cancer. There were "not bad" solid masses those damn spots could be. We were not there yet. And I honestly didn't go there yet. Things were spinning so fast I really didn't have time to look down. To me this was the hand of God walking me through the vertigo of it all, helping me out. I don't have any other way of explaining it. Someone much wiser once wrote about "a peace that passes understanding,"[11] which is about as close as I can come to describing it.

The next day Dr. Allen processed the findings with Dave and me. She also wanted to do one more diagnostic test, prior to the suggested invasive procedures. It's considered "alternative" and a bit controversial, but my experience with breast thermography was that it was a rather spot-on (pardon the pun) diagnostic weapon in the fight against breast cancer.[12] Basically, it's the use of infrared digital photography to capture the heat and blood flow in the breast. Apparently, cancer cells don't cool off like normal cells do. Climate control is key, therefore, in breast thermography.

Dr. Allen was meticulous in establishing the proper climate in the examination room, and in acclimating me to the climate of my discontent. It actually took most of Thursday to find just the right balance between the AC and the chill in my bones. Take one didn't quite work out. Although they'd winterized the room all morning, my low body temperature called for arctic measures. It took four more hours to put a proper chill in the air.

First, I had to take off my shirt and stand there, holding my hands above my head (to keep my arms from trying to trap some heat in my pits) while the technician took pictures. This was uncomfortable on many levels. But it got worse.

Next, I had to stick my hands in ice water and keep them submerged for what seemed like forever. I was so painfully cold that I almost started crying. I thought about the *Titanic*. Which didn't help. Because then I imagined my tears turning into icicles, dangling like stalactites from my cheek and chin. I decided I'd spell them *eye-cicles* if they did. That, actually, did help a teeny *t-eye-ny* bit.

Finally, Dr. Allen told me I could draw the ice cubes that used to be my hands out of the water. Then she told me to "put your hands up"—and *busted* is exactly how I felt, as I stepped back in front of the camera for mug shots of my breasts.

The digital images didn't bode well. There was no evidence of cooling. My fingers were still blue; my breasts looked red on the screen. In other words, my boobs were hot. I'm really not trying to brag. Just stating the facts.

---

[10] See the OUCH video by Geralyn Lucas at http://www.youtube.com/watch?v=yPXmEPBS75A

[11] Philippians 4:7

[12] http://www.huffingtonpost.com/christiane-northrup/the-best-breast-test-the-_b_752503.html

Chapter 4
I Was Too Sexy for My Shirt

Like I said, my boobs were hot.

Chapter 5
She's a Brick House

Well, Dr. Allen didn't exactly bust out The Commodores when she laid down the funk about my hot boobs.

She did say there was "definitely something going on" with my breasts, but, unfortunately, not in the happiest of ways. "It's not *definitely* cancer, but it is definitely *not* a healthy breast," is the way she put it.

Dave didn't like her frankness—on a couple of levels. (Besides the obvious, his sense of chivalry kicked in with all this dissing of my breasts. He was sticking up for my boobs. And don't think he wouldn't jump up on Dr. Allen's desk and belt out a little Lionel Richie in their defense. Because he totally would.)

I think I knew it was going to be cancer at this point, even though I wasn't swallowing let alone digesting it as a diagnosis, since it *wasn't* a diagnosis yet. Things had been happening so fast it felt like a dream sequence—but this was the first time I felt a pinch.

Even though she said it didn't necessarily, positively, mean cancer, Dr. Allen picked up the phone and booked me an appointment with Dr. Donna Stahl. *Cincinnati Magazine* had recently recognized her as one of Cincinnati's top doctors for 2007. I can't emphasize enough the ridiculous odds of me getting in to see her—the very next day. Superlatives aren't sufficient. If I had never felt God's hand on me before, there were fingerprints on my forehead—I felt them, but others seemed to sense them, too.

Dr. Allen told me that Dr. Stahl would probably schedule a biopsy and/or a possible excision at first. And, if things led to a recommended mastectomy and possible chemotherapy, she would support that aggressive medical course of action. I'm pretty sure she was pretty sure it was going to be cancer at that point, too.

I appreciated her rather un-composed candor. One would think that it all might have panicked me. I know Dave left her office not exactly feeling comforted. But for me, it was not mere brutal honesty, but more like truth that set me free[13]—*not* to panic, but to be prepared for whatever was to come.

I liked the way Dr. Stahl narrated as she performed a very thorough breast exam. She didn't exactly make direct references to "Brick House" either, but I did take note that she kept repeating the words "fatty tissue" over and over while examining my breasts.

I mention this solely for posterity's sake—for my boobs. (May they rest in peace.) They really were hot. And I just wanted to take this opportunity to document the true history of that medical fact, since it's not like I went around taking pictures of them to keep in a photo album on the coffee table. I didn't mention it in the dedication page, but this story is for them, too.

Dr. Stahl was encouraging. She said that we were hoping for a diagnosis of fibroadenoma, and scheduled a lumpectomy to remove and biopsy the damn spots. Then she sent me home to think "benign" thoughts over the weekend.

Dave and I left her office with high hopes and a couple of Western & Southern Financial Group Women's Open tickets I'd won at the tennis clinic earlier that week.

The license plate holder on my Mini says "Eat, Sleep, Tennis." I hadn't really done much of any of the above. Doctor visits had been filling my days instead of tennis. The damn spots were keeping me up at night because all I could think about was that *I just wanted them out!* As for the Eat part of the phrase, I refer back to the evidence already submitted in re: my very own, and I quote, "fatty tissue," to infer that my lack of appetite was merely a moot point.

Watching Amelie Mauresmo with her beautiful one-handed backhand was a delightful distraction. I got a little camera happy snapping photos of her backhand technique so I could study it and take notes for my own swing.

I didn't know that the following Tuesday was going to change everything. But I didn't think about that just then. I just enjoyed some good tennis, happily, and with some of my tennis girlfriends we ran into at the tournament. It's a night I will always remember as the last night I remember not having cancer.

Tuesday happened and all I knew was that it was five o'clock somewhere—and that somewhere was in the operating room where I was being prepped for a lumpectomy to excise and biopsy the three solid masses the tests had found in my left breast the week before. Unfortunately, it was five *a.m.* But still. Now, I don't remember saying any of this, but it seems in the twilight of my surgery I got quite chatty and a bit slaphappy and ordered a pinot grigio—from my breast surgeon. When I didn't hear any corks popping, I told Dr. Stahl that I would settle for a beer. Wrong five o'clock. As a last resort, I pleaded with the nurses to pretty please hook me up to a coffee IV so I wouldn't wake up with a headache. Unfortunately, the nearest Starbucks was in the lobby downstairs and everybody had already scrubbed up.

Dr. Stahl more than made up for thrice denying me beverage service in the operating room. It's almost like, for each time she had to say no to me, she removed one damn spot. Obviously, I completely forgave her, as I am told I kept telling her, "You rock!" Repeatedly. Over and over. Knowing me, I'm surprised I didn't try to get the wave going with the operating room staff. But knowing Dr. Stahl, that might have been a bit "over the top" and would have made her blush a little, so I doubt if she'd tell me if I did something like that. One of the cute things about awesome breast surgeons is how they are usually so busy being awesome and saving lives that they actually get caught off guard when you point out they are freaking superheroes.

The biopsy results wouldn't be available until the next day, but the pathologist told Dave the lumps looked "suspicious."

In a blog we were trying to keep updated for our out-of-town family members, Dave wrote, "We don't know if that meant they were wearing trench coats and dark sunglasses, or what?"[14]

Now it's probably obvious to you why we got married.

Our twisted humors are definitely one of the ways we cope. Our funny bones are connected.

But there is something else.

His next words were, "Whatever the outcome, we trust God. We pray that God will 'let this cup pass'[15] us by—but either way, we are going to keep loving each other, our kids, our family, our friends, our life and the Rock of our salvation."

It was pretty much the old "rock and a hard place" scenario. So I clung to the Rock. It steadied me somehow. Kept me from getting stirred. That's when it's five o'clock wherever I am. That's when it's time to sip on some comfort and cheer.

> "Though the mountains be shaken and the hills be removed, yet my unfailing love for you will not be shaken nor my covenant of peace be removed," says the LORD, who has compassion on you.[16]

I can't explain the comfort and cheer I received from drinking in those words, nor the peace that I experienced, even in that valley waiting for the phone call, except that Jesus loves me, this I know.

Knowing that, five o'clock or not, with or without a drink in my hand, is what I needed when I got the phone call.

---

[13] John 8:32

[14] http://www.blogintheshire.blogspot.com (September 2008-May 2010.)

[15] Matthew 26:39

[16] Isaiah 54:10

Chapter 6
I Don't Know Why

Dr. Stahl called me just before dinner. It was, actually, five o'clock. And that's truly not a cheap shot, or an attempt at being poetic even if my life is freaking poetic; it's just how the day played out. And boy, did I need a drink.

Pinot grigio, anyone? Yes, I had a pinot grigio. Or two. OK, maybe three. This happened to be one of those moments.

And the next time the clock struck five, I penned the following on my blogintheshire, which unfortunately got cancer when I did and turned into my cancer blog, where we posted updates for our friends and family:

> THURSDAY, AUGUST 21, 2008
> The Scoop
>
> I'm sorry it has taken until five a.m. to get to this blog update. I'm not going to lie—this is not the easiest blog to write. This has not been the easiest day. Parts of it have been lovely, though, so that's where I let myself drop at the end of the day, and that is where I find myself right now, sitting here, so I will start right there, if you don't mind, and then open the fortune cookie we got from the doctor today in proper form, after I've digested some of the day.

The Redheads and I hung tight and close to home all day, which is one of my favorite things. We all slept in for the first time since this whirlwind hit. The boys did not sleep the night before my surgery, and Amanda has been burning a candle at both ends with everything and her new job and beauty school. I think I may have just passed out from exhaustion. Or maybe it was the Vicodin. But the point is, sleeping in is also one of our favorite things, and a good way to start a day. Unless you have to be somewhere and you are late. Which occasionally happens in our home—but not today.

On days like today the things that matter most are crystal clear.

My mum and sister and nephew are here, so that's also nice to wake up to. I actually woke up to the lovely little pitter-patter of my nephew Brody's sweet feet, who apparently swept up with Olympic fervor, was in training for the hundred-yard dash around the race track that circles my dining room and kitchen. You really can't start training too early these days and I have to admire his dedication at two years old.

We all had a lovely picnic out on my back deck. My Redheads did a mini concert for us, which was the icing on top of lovely.

After lunch we watched a movie (Russell Crowe's *A Good Year*—uh, dramatic irony, anyone?) to pass the time before the phone call. We did not just sit around all day waiting for the phone call. We had a *really* good day, and then the phone call came.

Dave is out of town. I made him go ahead and go on his business trip because I didn't want to act like we were going to get bad news. He will be back tomorrow (Thursday) night.

That is how we are woven together.

I (had Mikeyy) conference Dave in, and the kids were right by my side, on speakerphone. The doctor said the damn spots were cancer. Grade 3, which is apparently aggressive. And if I understood the doctor correctly, the size of the three spots together was 2.3 centimeters. The one I had felt was very near the surface and she had to scrape to get what she could of it, but she couldn't get it all without taking some of my breast, which she didn't, obviously, at that time. But that's at least going to have to go. We have some big decisions to make this weekend before we meet with the doctor on Monday at five-thirty p.m. to discuss and jump into our game plan. We plan to be more aggressive than the cancer. I'm told I'm a wee bit competitive, so hopefully that's a good thing. We also need to go back and get some lymph nodes. And I think she mentioned chemo. Other than that, it was a fairly fuzzy phone call for me. It hit my Redheads hard and fast. Please pray for them anytime you think of me. I am not sure it has sunk into me yet, unless it is the pit that I have felt like throwing up since before dinner. But haven't. Yet.

This is me, shaken. To the core. In front of my kids. I don't know why.

I ordered the Redheads some pizza and some of my tennis girlfriends came over and we sat out on the back deck, drinking pinot grigio. Yeah, my girlfriends got my back. They B.Y.O.B.'d it, after they heard me sing "How Dry I Am" in the hospital. That's what girlfriends are for.

They also delivered P.F. Chang's to the Evanshire the night before, following my surgery. My cookie had a fantastic and apropos fortune in it that we are going with: good food brings health and longevity. Not to mention, the first lucky number mentioned is 42, which is my age. And I believe it is also a significant number for galaxy hitchhikers. Yes, I have the T-shirt; Mikeyy made me one for my forty-second birthday.

That's. Love. That's all I really know right now.

So that's the scoop. Thanks for praying.

That's where things were. And me, bookended there in the gift of the present.

We'd like to invite anyone who lives near to come over and pray with us Saturday night at seven as we'd like to bring out the big guns of prayer to begin this battle with and cast ourselves into our Father's very capable hands. And we go from there.

Hold my hand—sorry if it is shaking a little. Sometimes the sand moves fast. But isn't it so beautiful?

Posted by Joules Evans at 5:17 a.m.

Like I said, I had my three teenagers huddled around me when "the call" came. The doctor said the *C* word and it hit my kids hard. From my perspective it was as if that damn word had knocked my kids over. I don't remember breathing while I watched my kids succumb to the gravity of the moment as they fell to the ground. Literally. In three, separate sobbing heaps. Oh. My. Heart. Times three. Precious, shattered pieces on the floor. It was one of the most gut-wrenching mommy moments I've ever experienced. I desperately needed three laps and six arms right then. That's really all I was thinking about at that moment in time when it was standing *still* . . . like that.

That moment was the inciting incident in my life. It changed everything. Like September 11 changed everything. Like writing A.D. on the very first check after Jesus was born. Time had been counting down to that precise moment of PAX—the ground zero of history—then all of a sudden we're counting up.

I realize my inciting incident didn't have the same global implications. But that mommy moment became a hinge that held me fast, in the now. And I found some traction to do what I needed to do right then.

I stopped taking notes as soon as I wrote down the word that knocked my Redheads over and made them cry. I dropped the pencil that I'd drawn from behind my ear. I stopped listening to what Dr. Stahl was saying. I dropped the phone. There were no oxygen masks in the room anyway, and time had sort of stopped, so I dropped to the ground, gathered my precious babies, and rolled them up in my arms. That's how I stop, drop, and roll.

I did not process the fact that my doctor had just said I had cancer. Dave was still on the other end of the line with Dr. Stahl, processing everything. If it sounds horrible that he was out-of-town on a business trip that day, it really wasn't. He *had* cancelled the trip to stay home for "the call" but like I said, I told him it would be like expecting the worst if he stayed. So he went, for me. I made him go. I needed him to go. Now I needed him to stay on the phone with my doctor. When I stopped, dropped, and rolled, he picked up the ball. Thank God. There was no time for him to stop, drop, and roll. There were more words to listen to, more notes to take, questions to ask, appointments to schedule, research to be done, decisions to be made, tears to cry, groans to be uttered, prayers to be prayed, a plane to catch, a sickly wife and three grief-stricken kids to come home to, phone calls to make, a business to run, insurance forms to fill out, dinner to be picked at, insomnia to be had, pieces of our world to pick up, after of course he finished this phone call, knowing there was no time to go look in the mirror and see what he was made of. That's just how he rolls, when I stop, drop, and roll.

And that's how we roll.

I don't know why Dr. Stahl had to say the *C* word. I do know that sometimes words do hurt, though. No matter what people say about sticks and stones. Or rock, paper, scissors for that matter. Words beat them all.

I don't know how I got cancer. Damn spot.

I didn't know where all this was going to lead. Were my days about to begin counting down?

All I knew was my children might lose their mother.

I don't know why.

All I knew was I loved them.

And all I could think about was right now. Right here. So I held them fast, like I wouldn't let go.

Meanwhile, my mom and Jennie were downstairs in the family room, flipping channels and magazine pages, fielding phone calls, folding my laundry, imagining doors opening, straining ears for footsteps, watching ice melt in their Diet Cokes while clocking Brody's laps, wishing the clock would keep up with him, waiting for someone to come tell them what the doctor had said. The glasses weren't the only ones sweating.

Jennie summed it up like this:

> Mom and I were sitting in the living room at my sister's house, waiting desperately for someone to emerge from upstairs with news from the call. In a moment that seemed to stand still *forever*, Amanda quietly walked downstairs to where we were. My heart went to pieces as she looked at me and then just fell broken into my arms. It felt like all the oxygen left the room when I realized that my sister had breast cancer. Amanda and I fell into a sobbing heap, onto the loveseat. Mom began hyperventilating the second we heard the *C* word. I don't know how she managed to make it across the room, but she fell onto the loveseat, becoming part of the heap with us. She and I sandwiched Amanda. We all felt like we were drowning, and all we could do was hold on to each other.

Chapter 7
Mother and Child Reunion
(The Redheads—In Their Own Words)

Before you slam the book shut...the following picture is not what you may think. My sweet children were not flipping me off nor did I choose this photo to flip you, dear reader, off. Rather, on the way to Racing for a Cure for their mum, Amanda got that very finger slammed in the door of our minivan, who goes by the name Yukon. We almost had to change route and race to the hospital. But once Amanda caught her breath and could wiggle and "flip" her finger, she decided it really said what she felt, both in that moment, and even more appropriately, about her mum getting cancer. She asked me to take a picture, and the boys quickly stood proudly with their "little" sister: such sweet solidarity amongst siblings. This picture means more to me than you can imagine. And with that, I'd like to introduce my Redheads.

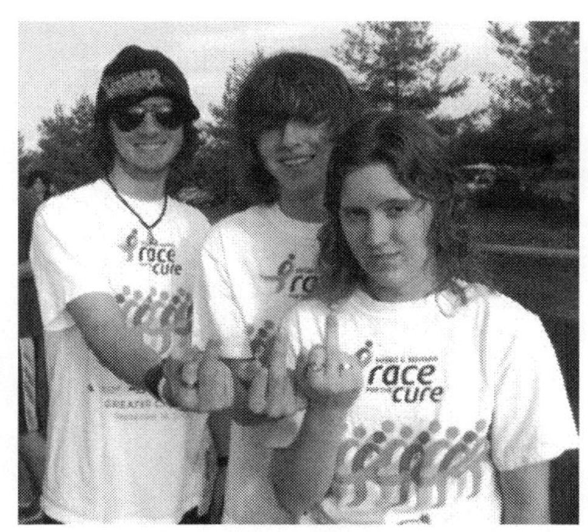

Amanda at 17 years old

Legends and stories often have more to do with shaping a culture or person than the actuality behind those stories. I like this—I think it's true. Please, don't take the following as the word of God, but rather as the discombobulated memories of a girl. The facts here may have been entirely made up.

There is a tremor that runs through this memory—as an earthquake in my brainwaves. We all gathered in my brother Matt's bedroom. My dad was on speakerphone—he was away somewhere. The doctor was on a different speaker. Gravity was unsure of what to do. The air felt unsteady and wobbled like a depressive drunk. I think it had grown thicker, too, possibly to catch me when I heard what it somehow already knew.

I don't know what the doctor said. I don't even remember the doctor's gender. The only distinct thing that I remember is the sound of an implosion—and then the feeling of being submerged. It felt as though my spinal cord had been snapped and my brain set afloat in the stormy sea of cerebrospinal fluid. I think of the execution of Nicholas II, the last Russian tsar: a family lined up and murdered—shot. My brothers broke. My mum instantly became mortal. My Dad, though . . . In my memory, there was an audible creaking—as though his spine was an ancient tree being straightened out. A groaning—as though he were a wooden ship being stressed from too much weight. A thump—as this new load, *in sickness*, dropped on him: the sound of a man becoming Atlas.

I walked away from the room, only able to stand because of the air's thickness pillowing around me. Everything felt loosened and unconnected as I treaded downstairs to the couch. Be the adult, now—that's what I was thinking.

I walked up to my Aunt Jennie. So far, so strong. But as I tried to force the word *cancer* out of my mouth, I found myself to be broken too. Collapsed. Aunt Jennie's arms gathered me up, and I remember resting against her breasts. I felt as though I were merely a page in a book and the epitome's cover slammed heavily against me.

We wept.

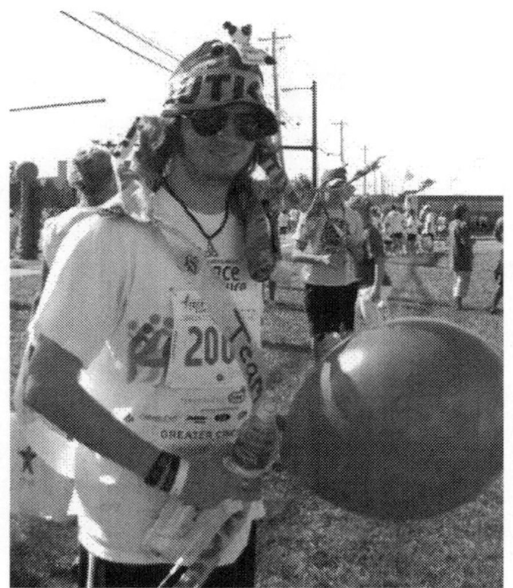

Matt at 15 years old

The whole day was a really big blur. I remember it seemed like it moved so fast, but at the same time it was also one of the slowest days ever. Mikeyy and I had been in my room playing Portal on our Xbox 360 for the previous couple of days, like going through the portals in the game took us through a portal out of our lives for just a bit. It seemed like the best thing to do to keep our minds off of everything going on. Then I just remember all of us in my room, huddled around the phone. Trying to get the phone conference going seemed like it took hours. The doctor's voice had no real emotion, which just made it all the scarier. Finally, we got everyone on the phone: Dad conferenced in with us and the doctor. I don't think any of us breathed the whole time the doctor was talking. Nothing she said made any sense to me. My mum was healthy. Nothing was wrong with her. Everything was fine. But then I was sitting there and the doctor was saying she had cancer. Then it hit me. I remember thinking about how ever since I was little, whenever Dad would leave on business trips, he would tell me that while he was gone, I was the man of the house. It eventually just became second nature so that he didn't even have to tell me. I didn't think I should cry because Dad was gone, which made me the man of the house. I didn't think the man of the house would cry—I cried anyway though. I remember sitting in the corner by my bedroom door holding Amanda and Mikeyy. None of us really knew what to do. What can you do in that kind of a situation? I went and sat in my closet. Something about the dark enclosed space of my closet always makes me feel safe.

Mum picked the phone back up and she, Dad and the doctor stayed on for a while longer. I just kind of sat there in shock. Our whole lives had been shaken and everything was different. Everything seemed dark and rainy and just downright sucky then but I never even thought about the silver lining that would come.

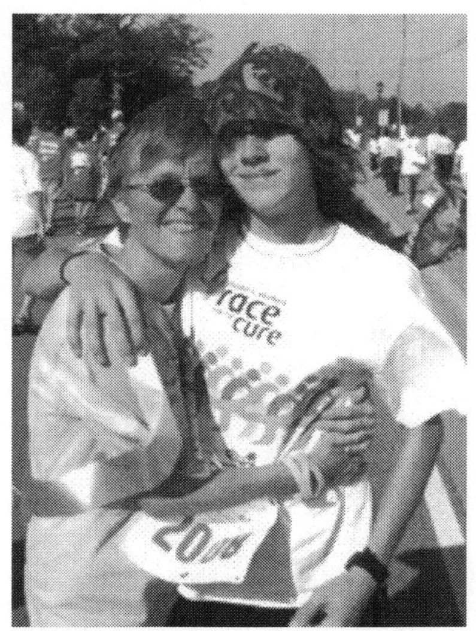

Mikeyy at 14 years old

I don't cry a lot. In fact, I only cried once throughout the whole cancer earthquake that shook our world. I didn't even cry once throughout the entire film, *The Notebook*. If you were to bottle up all the tears I shed year-round to give water to people in Nigeria, you would not even provide one person with 1/24th of the water needed in a day. If my tears were Noah's flood, Noah would only be the size of seven molecules bonded together. In fact, eighty percent of the time water drops from my eyes, it's my body rushing to my aid whenever I engage in my staring contest addiction, or me staring till I fake cry, so that Mum's sweet little heart wants to give me whatever I want. That, or I'm just tired.

A time without tears can actually be a sad time. I've found throughout my life that when sad instances come along, tears are a little inadequate when it comes to expressing how I feel.

This instance was no different.

I did not cry when we got the phone call. I did not cry when we all dropped to the floor. I did not cry when the realization sunk in that I might not have my mum around much longer. I did not cry.

Like I said, crying did not seem adequate in a situation like this. Instead, I nothing-ed. Nothing-ing seemed a little more appropriate. It at least made sense. Nothing I said or did would change anything. Nothing I felt would fix this. Nothing leaving my eyes would help. So I felt nothing—nothing but despair.

Chapter 8
Wish I Could Save You

The next day when Dave got back in town, we gathered around our summer dining table out on the back deck and tried to collect ourselves. I don't remember what we ate, or if we ate, for that matter. But we did lay all our cards on the table: Dave, Amanda, Matt, Mikeyy, and me.

The lumps Dr. Stahl had removed were in a clump that measured 2.3 centimeters. The initial lump, the damn spot I had found, was in the "milky way" duct. The cancer was classified as an invasive ductile carcinoma (grade 3: very aggressive and fast growing). It had already begun spreading and had left the duct and invaded the breast. We didn't know if it had reached the lymph nodes or anywhere else yet. We would not know the stage of the cancer until those cards were played.

The pathology report confirmed that the cancer was both ER and PR negative, which meant it couldn't be treated with hormonal therapy like tamoxifen. But it was HER2 positive—*finally*, something positive—amplified even (6.2, which apparently is *quite* positive). That meant it *could* be treated with immunotherapy, such as Herceptin. I had a cancer type that *used to be* a death sentence—before Herceptin. In 2005, *The New England Journal of Medicine* published clinical trial reports that found Herceptin to reduce the risk of relapse in breast cancer patients by fifty percent when given after breast cancer surgery, before the cancer has spread, and after chemotherapy, for one year.[17] This was going to be a very long, very hard ordeal. But Herceptin felt like an ace up my sleeve.

Dr. Stahl had told us that she wasn't happy with the margins the lumpectomy left. The damn spot had been attached to the surface (the nipple of the milky way, if that's not TMI) so we would definitely have to go back and take the rest of it. She recommended a double mastectomy and the removal and biopsy of five lymph nodes—then we would know the stage of the cancer—followed by chemotherapy. That was my medical option. Go bold or go home.

Reconstruction was not on the table at that point. Dr. Stahl said not until after chemo. I was relieved, actually, to have this decision out of my hands. The pressure I felt over that particular option stressed me out. I had no idea if I wanted to play the reconstruction card or not. It would mean more surgeries and more recovery time at a time when my Redheads were spreading their wings and about to fly the Evanshire. Having boobs didn't seem to rate when compared to spending my time with my Redheads. I didn't mind Dr. Stahl removing the reconstruction card from the deck so I could stop sweating about it. Although, come to think of it, sweating (but especially freezing) in my tennis outfit would be way less embarrassing without nipples always "pointing" out the obvious.

None of the five of us had a very good poker face when it came to dealing with cancer. There was no bluffing my Redheads. When we began homeschooling sixteen years ago, the mother of the family we homeschooled with, my dear friend Sue, was diagnosed with breast cancer. She had a lumpectomy but chose not to pursue the traditional medical route beyond that. During the initial frenzy of research we plunged into after Sue's diagnosis, we had come across *A Cancer Battle Plan*, by David and Anne Frahm and *The Hallelujah Diet*, by George Malkmus. I remember reading them and thinking what a daunting, full-time job fighting cancer seemed like. I was overwhelmed, for Sue. Sue, however, was undaunted. The second she put the books down, she put up her dukes and came out fighting.

Sue sought out a naturopath to help plot and supervise her cancer battle plan, which included an intensive detox and complete overhaul of her diet and lifestyle. The day I met Sue, one of the first things I learned about her was that she was seriously addicted to Dr Pepper and M&M's. She didn't say anything; I could just tell. The day she started her cancer battle plan, Sue kicked both habits, cold turkey. And never looked back. Of course, that wasn't the entirety of her cancer battle plan, but it is one of my favorite memories of her.

She fought valiantly, gracefully, successfully, for seven years, until the breast cancer came back with a vengeance, having gone to her lymph nodes, liver, and lungs. She continued to fight valiantly, gracefully, for the rest of her life.

We walked through her first cancer battle with her, every step of the way, even to the point of making similar (though not to the full extent) dietary and lifestyle choices. For us, they were choices. For Sue, they were life and death. I made those choices with my friend because I would have followed the same cancer battle plan back then.

I have to admit, besides being utterly grief-stricken, I was also entirely disillusioned when Sue died. I remember standing by her coffin, saying goodbye and telling her I would miss her. I remember taking it out on my juicer the next day by throwing it away.

My kids remembered cancer.

I could practically see them doing the math in their heads: 2008 + S-E-V-E-N years = 2015, to spell it out—because nobody dared to say that number out loud. But everybody was thinking it. You could read it on all of our faces just as plainly as if we all had the seven of spades stuck to our foreheads.

My kids *begged* me to follow Dr. Stahl's medical advice.

I knew it was tearing them up inside seeing their mum face cancer. I wished I could save them from that. I knew Dave wished he could just take it all away. I wished I wasn't cashing in my *in sickness* chips. I wished I could save him from the *for worse* part that was at hand.

I knew they all wished they could save me.

I knew I wouldn't give up till it was over.

If I had to have an aggressive type of cancer, we'd just have to try and be even more aggressive than the cancer. Dr. Stahl agreed that this was the best chance to make the cancer fold, even if it meant raising the stakes that high. They were pretty high already. It wasn't a choice really. It was life or death.

Having laid our cards, face-up, on the table, we called Dr. Stahl and scheduled to have the breasts that I had nursed my babies with cut off my body on August 29, 2008, so I could keep being my kids' mum. It really was as simple as that.

Then Dave cancelled the Caribbean getaway we'd previously booked to celebrate our twentieth anniversary. We'd kept the trip planned up to this point because we hoped. We hoped I did not have cancer. We hoped I would be able to continue healing from the lumpectomy at the cute little purple beach house that we'd rented on Grand Cayman Island. They didn't have to, but the generous souls who owned the house gave us a full refund and wished me well, saying they hoped that we would re-book someday.

Time will tell, but odds are good that this pair will someday play our cards right: full house, jokers wild.

---

[17] http://www.nejm.org/doi/full/10.1056/NEJMoa052306#t=article

Chapter 9
That I May Live

People ask me all the time if I ever went around asking God "Why me?" when I found out I had cancer.

Before I got cancer, I spent much of my life being a rather introspective sort with a melancholic bent, who would have had no trouble at all coming up with a hundred reasons why me. In a way, cancer kind of cured me of that by shaking my black bile silly, to the point of having the gall to wash the bitter down with something sweet.

Like when I was a kid and I would trick my mouth into swallowing peas whenever my mom ruined my plate by piling on those nasty green balls of mush. I *still* don't like peas. These days, the closest I get to peas is when I'm picking them out of basmati rice at Indian restaurants. Honestly, I don't get the whole aesthetic argument. Green is one of my favorite colors, but peas are *not* attractive. They are mushy. I used to have a T-shirt with a funny cartoon and caption that said, "If your mom tries to give you peas, just say no." I could have used that shirt when I was a kid, when my mom made me eat peas despite my pleas and promises that I would for sure throw up. She was not moved. So before she threatened to scoop on more peas, I'd take a big swig of Kool-Aid and tip my head back like I was going to gargle. But instead of gargling, I would drop a single pea into the swirl of the grape gully and try to wash it down without actually making contact with the pea, until it splashed down into my stomach acid. Then I would rinse and repeat until my plate was clean and my mom stopped rolling her eyes at me.

I should probably say thank you to my mom for the useful strategy, not to mention the cool analogy. (I'd like to clarify that I'm not exactly saying thanks for the peas, though.)

When you find out that you have cancer, there's not much you can do about it. I just lifted my glass, said "Cheers!" in as many languages as I could Google, prayed for my health, and tried to swallow the *C* word like I had swallowed all those nasty peas.

There are, however, some "peas" I don't even try to swallow.

When little kids get cancer, I do wonder why. When my friend Sue died from cancer, I did wonder why. When I hear of somebody getting cancer practically every time I turn around these days, I do wonder why.

I don't know why. The truth is, this shakes me more than my own cancer did. I had to wrap my head around my own cancer, and then put my dukes up. There is no wrapping my head around somebody else's cancer.

It. Just. Never. Makes. Sense.

And watching someone else have to go through cancer breaks my heart. To an extent I can empathize, but I can only imagine what it's like to be in *their* shoes. They are the ones who have to wear them and I know from experience they are quite heavy.

When I got cancer, my shoes got heavy. Partly because of the gravity of the *C* word, partly because of the grievous thought of not being around for my kids' lives, partly because of the soul searching that I assume is par for the course when facing one's mortality, and partly because my feet literally got, and still are a bit, soggy from the chemo. Cancer shook me like I've never been shaken and the truth is I don't know how I'm still standing, except the grace of God, by which I stand—soggy feet and all.[18]

Shaken, all we could do was fall to our knees and ask God to heal me, that I may live.

Dave had been spending some time reading *The Message*, seeking counsel and a little comfort and cheer. He found that he especially connected with the battle strategy of King Jehoshaphat.

Jehoshaphat had just received a report that there was a huge force on its way to fight him, and there was no time to waste. Then it says,

"Shaken, Jehoshaphat prayed."[19] Jehoshaphat's people came from all the cities around and that's just what they did. Dave felt the parallels were as rich as they were ridiculous cool, so he decided to keep in step with Jehoshaphat's battle plan. After all, it had turned out so well for Jehoshaphat and his people that they all ended up in a place called the Valley of Blessing.

I know Dave was shaken and felt helpless in the face of my cancer. It's a pretty huge enemy. So we prayed. And all our friends came over to pray with us.

We looked to God.

We believed it was God's war, not ours.

We were hoping God would heal me.

We asked him to heal me. Boldly, we begged.

I can't tell you how beautiful and humbling it was to have my kids laying hands on me, begging God to heal their mum that I may live. We were in the middle of our living room floor and there were layers and layers of friends laying hands on us all, praying for us all. And that was how we began our cancer battle plan.

Then, Dave popped in one of our favorite CDs, serendipitously entitled *Remedy*, and slowly people started singing along. At first, it was difficult finding our voices through the emotion and the tears. But when we got to the chorus of "You Never Let Go" something let loose and we were louder than the music. The only words to describe how it felt to have everyone literally crying out for me like that, in chorus, would be: *lifted up*.

I cast myself into the arms of Our Father who is in heaven[20] that night and I haven't looked back. What else was there to do but put one foot in front of the other like I'm headed for tomorrow, believing God is with me? It doesn't really hurt anyone if I'm wrong and it doesn't work. But what if I'm not?

That prayer meeting was on August 23, 2008—which also happened to be Dave's forty-third birthday. Some birthday, I know. Poor guy. I was so busy recovering from the lumpectomy and the shock from hearing the *C* word that I didn't even think to plan a birthday party. Dave had been equally preoccupied: plotting our cancer battle plan, praying that God would heal me, hoping that I may live, wondering if he may lose his wife . . . too busy to even remember it was his birthday. Neither of us can remember if there was a birthday cake or if he blew out any candles. I think I know what his wish was, though.

Unfortunately, there were a couple of "bumps" in the road, which I knew he would be super sad to see removed, on the way to that wish come true, not to mention more birthdays.

---

[18] Romans 5:2

[19] 2 Chronicles 20:3 (MSG)

[20] Matthew 6:9–13

Chapter 10
Man, I Feel Like a Woman

Sure, the optimist can say the cup is half full when it *is* half full, but what about when both "cups" are about to be empty?

So what did I do to mentally prepare myself to go in and have my breasts cut off?

It's not like I think I can dance with the stars or anything, but I just tried putting one foot in front of the other. What I ended up with was some clumsily choreographed mash-up kind of a dance—something between a two-step and a waltz, with a little bit of a hip-*hope* groove just to shake things up.

Step 1: I went out with the girls and let my hair down. Literally. To the ground. As in, I got it cut off. Well, not all the way off. But I did get a new haircut. I was told that after my mastectomy it would be a while before I could raise my hands above my head, and since I am a quick thinker, I thought, "Whoa, I wonder how I'll shampoo my hair?" Clip. Problem solved.

Honestly, I probably learned this idea from Matt when he was four years old and sitting at his desk one day, learning to read. I was doing math with Amanda, and I could hear Matt getting a little frustrated about something. I just assumed it was over blending consonants, and I was trying to wrap up with Amanda so I could give him my full attention. All of a sudden I heard a clip, and then,

"That's better." I looked over and Matt's bangs were blurring the letters on the page he was "reading" in his *Teach Your Child to Read in 100 Easy Lessons* book. Matt's bright green preschool scissors were sitting on top of the pile of bangs like they were trying to make some kind of a point . . . which I got. Now it was my turn to try to blend in his new 'do.

It took me a while to get used to me with a boy cut. But it really shouldn't have surprised me with the spy ops training I had done in my youth. Disguises 101. Duh.

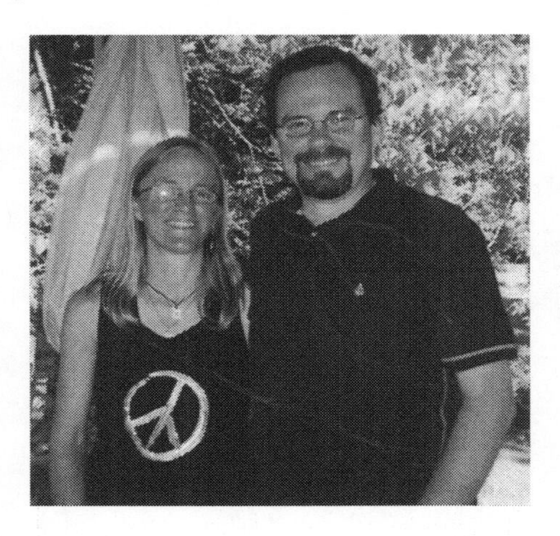

That summer my hair was the longest it had been since I got tired of sitting on my hair in second grade and had it lopped off to my shoulders. I don't think I'm blowing my own cover at this point, now that it's a moot one, to hint that one of my aliases had to do with a certain little girl of fairy tale lore who hung out with bears. I can't say how many bears there were because that is classified. Suffice it to say that my hair used to be down past my shoulders and it was dirty dishwater blonde. I know what they say about blondes and all, but I was about to be bald shortly. I didn't feel like missing out on any fun. I didn't feel like taking any chances. I just decided go with Shania on this one and exercise my "prerogative to have a little fun." So I grabbed a few girlfriends and we turned a salon and a haircut into a party. I also definitely channeled a little Cindy Lauper, even if my true color would soon be shining through—like a cue ball.

How cool was it that my stylist that day "happened" to have gone through this very similar chemotherapy 'do transition scene with her own mum, who was a sixteen-year breast cancer survivor, now seventy-five years old! Coincidence? Well, what would be the fun in that? I know this may be totally politically incorrect, but I just can't help but believe it was a God moment.[21] I like to play connect the dots between moments like these and imagine the outline of the hand of God that the big picture will reveal someday.

Step 2: I couldn't really sidestep pre-op testing, even though it meant a few more needle sticks. One jab that hurt the most was when they told me I couldn't have a glass of wine with my dinner the night before my surgery. That just seemed a little "over the top." If it's five o'clock anywhere, it's definitely five o'clock wherever I'm at the night before my mastectomy. I totally appealed that order, and after being forwarded so many times even I'd consider my message spam, I got permission for one measly glass of wine, from some nurse or best friend or second cousin of a nurse, who said she was tight with my anesthesiologist, who said it was okeydokey with him. Whew.

Step 3: The night before my mastectomy I went to another prayer meeting the Redheads' youth pastor Alton had organized for three high-school students' mothers, all of whom were in critical situations. Yott's mother was waiting on a lung transplant. Theresa Maria's mother was having brain surgery at the same time I was having my mastectomy. I was the only mum who was physically able to attend. I didn't even know the other mothers at that point. But I prayed for them from that night forward, when we three were joined together and lifted up by our kids. To me, without this step, it would be like trying to dance with two left feet.

Step 4: (A little to the left now.) My tennis girlfriends and I let it all hang out and had a bra burning.

Which somehow seems "fitting" since the event fell on the same evening of Obama's address at the Democratic National Convention. I'm not sure if it's politically correct to say that, either. But then again we were burning bras, and I'm pretty sure I've already crossed the line plenty anyhow. I don't mean to get out of line so much. It's just that I never really learned to dance.

And have I mentioned that the bras I was burning were *brand new* ones I had just bought at Victoria's—or is that a Secret? But seriously, I can't remember the last time I had bought a bra prior to that. Although, now, I will always remember the *last* time I ever bought one. (And good riddance, in a way—if you know what I mean.)

So I finally decide to buy new bras—a *month* before I get diagnosed with breast cancer and have to have an emergency double mastectomy. It literally took me five hours to get fitted and find the cup that was "just right."

Timing is everything.

Dramatic irony happens. I like it when I can find a way to laugh about it. I'd way rather laugh about it than kick myself in the ass for buying expensive bras I'm just going to toss into a bonfire.

It wasn't exactly a burning bush—more like a barbeque pit—but my girlfriends and I all tossed in bras. I threw in the brand-spanking new bra I had barely worn but couldn't bear to return empty, as it were. My friend Heidi threw in a box of Band-Aids, which we all got a huge kick out of. They were BIG Band-Aids after all (wink, wink). It was truly one of those *Divine Secrets of the Ya-Ya Sisterhood* types of moments, which I will never ever forget.

Step 5: And now, for the bow, thanks for the mammaries, I mean, memories. In other words, it was *the* Kodak moment—for my boobs, for posterity, for my hubby. Hey, every guy is a breast man, right? Well I thought Dave ought to have a postcard or two, so sue me, but I had my sister, who happens to be a professional photographer, take a few pictures.

Unfortunately, my computer crashed before I had the guts to get the pictures developed for him. We may never know, but we suspect that it wasn't just my shirt that I was too sexy for—but the whole world. And especially my poor computer, which, after that particular upload was no longer PC.

Curtain Call: I packed my bags for the hospital, took a Valium, and then it was curtains for me. I went to sleep, resting in God, and woke up still there. Then we piled into Yukon (affectionately named after our favorite blend of Starbucks coffee, which sort of irked me in my de-caffeinated state) and headed off to the hospital.

What else was there to do? With the prospect of both "cups" soon to be empty, all I knew to do was to trust the one who was pouring. Somehow, he makes even empty cups overflow.

---

[21] C. S. Lewis called them *Thin Places.*

Chapter 11
Fix You

It was *exactly* the same kind of buzzer they give you at P.F. Chang's.

Except, when you're at P.F. Chang's and the lights start flashing, you've hit the jackpot. You know in that salivating Pavlovian way that Lettuce Wraps—Lettuce Wraps—Lettuce Wraps are soon to be your good fortune.

When the buzzer goes off in the pre-op waiting room, you know you are going to be lucky to get ice chips.

I was already grumpy because I was worried that I would wake up from my surgery with a caffeine headache. I know, that's the last thing you'd expect someone to be thinking about before her mastectomy, but there it is. I was.

I had a cup of coffee around ten p.m. at the bra burning, sort of, as a preventive measure. It was Folgers. Somebody laced it with a bit of chocolate, but I knew it was Folgers. (I may be a bit of a coffee snob, but I hope I am not rude when someone is nice enough to brew me a cup of coffee. Practically any cup of coffee somebody else brews for me is always "good to the last drop" if you ask me.) So I drank it with a happy heart.

But I was worried if the jolt was going to be enough to get me to the other side of my surgery.

The other last thing you might expect to hear about before my mastectomy is that Dave and I had a fight upon waking up, at the butt crack of dawn, in the midst of getting ready to hop in Yukon and head to the hospital.

I don't remember what the fight was about. I called my hubby while I was writing this chapter, and he can't remember what it was about either. I blame my memory lapse on chemo. I think Dave is just forgetful. Which has been quite helpful, I'm sure, in putting up with all my shenanigans all these years.

Knowing us, it was most likely something ridiculous—like his coffee breath. Which, in retrospect, I can imagine would've only added insult upon Yukon's previous insult to my perceived injury that was percolating in me due to lack of caffeine. Once, Dave and I fought over whether to keep the thermostat at seventy-seven or seventy-eight degrees—that's how ridiculous our arguments can be. I'm still ridiculous enough to stand by that extra degree I got all steamed over. I'm pretty sure Dave thinks he's Mr. Cool and not ridiculous at all, that he still stands by depriving me that degree of warmth.

We did make up before we got to the hospital.

I honestly don't remember a whole lot about my mastectomy.

I remember the surgery waiting room receptionist giving me the P.F. Chang's buzzer and I remember doing my little shtick about it.

I remember a bunch of people I love showing up and filling the surgery waiting room area.

I remember my buzzer going off and the main thing that was alarming me at that point was getting the IV put in. I like getting IVs way less than I like peas.

Once I was appropriately attired and the IV was in place, I remember everyone packing into my room to pray for me before they rolled me into the operating room.

I had asked one of my pastors, Dan Henry, to bring me communion just in case they would let me take it before going into surgery. Just in case, if you know what I mean. He brought me communion in his backpack. Which he placed on the gurney by my feet and unzipped, revealing to me a holy grail and some bread from heaven. Of course I wasn't allowed to partake. All I can say is, we tried. And, when somebody tries to smuggle me communion before my surgery, it ranks way up there with people who make me coffee.

Thanks, Dan. Besides, I channeled my inner Peter Pan and took it anyway—in my imagination. Or maybe I'm just stubborn?

I remember my kids' youth pastor, Alton, taking over my shtick to lighten the mood. He practically had the room in stitches, which I thought seemed fair, all things considered. Plus, I was wishing they would start the happy gas already. It was good having a little comic relief. Thanks, Alton.

I remember right before they rolled me back that everybody began to lay hands on me to pray over me. But not everybody fit in the room, so there were layers of people laying hands on me and each other, and spilling out into the hallway.

I don't remember being scared. One of my tennis girlfriends, an oncology nurse, had given me a worry stone with the words, "Perfect love casts out all fear"[22] etched on it. I hung on to that, literally, and in every way imaginable.

As they rolled me into the operating room I wondered if I would say anything funny while under this time. I remember asking Dr. Stahl to let me know if I did so I could add it to my repertoire.

I remember they stretched my arms out which made me think of Jesus.

I'm not bringing that up because I'm trying to make myself into a Christ figure in this story. I don't have a Christ complex. Though I do want to be like him.

It wasn't exactly green pastures that I was lying down in.[23] Still, the happy juice started flowing in my IV.

It might have been the valley of the shadow of death, but somehow the thought of him comforted me.

I remember waking up in the recovery room and feeling like I didn't really know what dying of thirst was before that moment. The recovery room was packed, and my nurse was like a pinball in my periphery, trying to keep up with caring for two other patients. One poor patient was hurling in the bed right next to me. I know it's horrible, but I immediately felt sorry for myself. See, I'm a sympathetic puker. I wondered if it was possible to accidentally turn inside out while retching, without a drop of spit to help lubricate things. The other poor patient was having some colorectal issues in the bed kitty-corner from me. I recognized that my need for an ice chip, or especially a kind face was understandably pretty low on the totem pole, but I was totally feeling sorry for myself anyway. My eyes welled up with tears and I wondered where in the world they came from, because I sure was thirsty.

Yep, I had just had a mastectomy, but I was crying like a baby—over an ice chip.

I knew the P.F. Chang's buzzer was a bad idea.

Even in the midst of her whirlwind, my nurse noticed the first tear erupt. I don't think she even knew I was awake before the tears started dropping. When our eyes met she immediately came over to my bed to wipe it off, gave me the kind smile I needed, some kind words, and even ice chips.

Then she had to resume her pinball game.

What I remember about the rest of my recovery room experience is that it consisted of me watching the minute hand of the clock on the wall, while praying the Lord's Prayer for an hour and a half solid, so I wouldn't hear the hurling sounds next to me. I tried to rotate in the Nicene Creed, but I kept messing it up and I got mad at myself about that. Which I didn't think was very productive, so I just kept with the Lord's Prayer.

And I remember the cup of coffee my tennis buds brought me the morning after my mastectomy. I *so* needed that caffeine fix. And I'm not going to lie—the blueberry scone just about brought tears to my eyes.

I don't really remember much else from my mastectomy.

I know I lost something that I can't replace, but I just remember that Dr. Stahl tried to fix me.

---

[22] 1 John 4:18

[23] Psalm 23

Chapter 12
Be OK

It rained on the day of my mastectomy, as if the clouds understood the gravity of my situation and had quite a pity party for me.

I didn't hear the rain. But all the people I love who were sitting in the waiting room heard it.

My daughter Amanda told me she tried not to cry. She said she knew that if she started, she wouldn't be able to stop. So instead, she and her friend Kiley left the waiting room and decided the only thing left to do was to go dance in the rain for a little while.

That's my baby girl.

My sister Jennie also told me she tried not to cry. But at the sight of everyone laying hands on me and each other and spilling out into the hallway, her dam burst.

It's possible that this is what really set the clouds off.

A kind nurse gave her a Kleenex and some kind words. That means a lot to me, since I wasn't able to be there for her while she was trying to be there for me.

Oh my heart.

Here's what was going on in Jennie's:

> All I knew was that my sister needed to be OK. I flew in from Charleston to be there for her double mastectomy. The day I got there I happened to find a four-leaf clover in her front yard. I told her that there had to be an Irish angel named Rachel watching over her. Rachel was an Irish friend and roommate of mine who died in a tragic car accident a few years ago. The four-leaf clover made me think of Rachel. For some reason, that made me feel like everything was going to be OK.
>
> At the hospital, we all gathered around Joules's bed. That room was so packed. The family stood right at her side as people laid hands upon hands on Joules, and us, and each other, on and on, out into the hallway. It was something like out of a movie. The intensity of the love that filled the room and all the prayers overwhelmed me so much. There were waves of prayers, even as there were waves of people. I wanted to say a prayer too, but I kept getting caught in the waves. And especially the waves of my own tears. I was so scared, not knowing what was going to happen to Joules, that I couldn't stop crying. I was beside myself, desperate for those prayers to work. As I left the room, I was having a hard time catching my breath from crying. I guess I was hyperventilating. One of the nurses took me by the hand and guided me into a quiet room, where she sat me down and tried to calm me down. She gave me a warm wet towel and put her arm around my shoulder. She reminded me to breathe. Once I caught my breath, I collected myself and headed to the waiting room with the rest of the group.

I know both my baby sister and my baby girl needed me to be OK.

I know everybody in the waiting room wanted to know that I'd be OK.

My friend Debbie brought some pieces of fabric to the waiting room. She wanted people to write messages to me on them, to help pass the time. This was a divine distraction, especially for Dave, who, as I've explained, is not easily distracted when it comes to double doors coming between us.

What he remembers of the time in the waiting room was focusing on finding the perfect Bible verse to write on his small white piece of fabric. If you have ever played Scrabble with him, you know how his turn is always a convenient time to get in some good reading, say, dig a little deeper into Dante's *Divine Comedy* (complete and unabridged, in Italian) once whistling the *Jeopardy* song gets old. Seriously, you can actually hear the gears cranking as he methodically, *painstakingly*, goes through *every* possible combination of tiles/letters/words/plays before he will TAKE HIS FREAKING TURN ALREADY! (Sorry about that . . . just writing about it makes me feel like I'm stranded in a flashback in front of my tile rack, with my next word all ready whenever I make it through *Purgatario* this turn. I am also acutely aware that part of his meticulous process involves trying to checkmate my intended spot on the board. But I digress.) The point is, that while Dave twirled his felt-tip pen around his knuckles the way he does, and thumbed through the Bible trying to find the perfect verse to write on his piece of fabric, I think it's fair to say that I descended into and emerged from the *Inferno* of my mastectomy.

Debbie later took all the pieces of fabric and wove them together. She framed them with gerbera daisies and made a beautiful quilt for me. Appropriately, the colors of the quilt are black and white, with bright LIVESTRONG yellow accents.

I feel like those messages—and the earlier prayers—covered me.

They cover me still, every time I wrap up in that warm but oh-so-cool quilt.

And since inquiring minds want to know, the verse Dave chose was 1 Peter 5:9-11:

> So keep a firm grip on the faith. The suffering won't last forever. It won't be long before this generous God who has great plans for us in Christ—eternal and glorious plans they are—will have you put together and on your feet for good. He gets the last word; yes, he does.

I know, P-E-R-F-E-C-T on a triple word score, right? There is, after all, a method to his madness.

Finally, Dr. Stahl came out into the waiting room and debriefed my peeps on Operation Fix Me.

You might be thinking of the opening scene of *The Bionic Woman* as you read this part. And that is fine with me. There is an awful lot of truth in fiction, and I'd just like to leave it at that.

No, I did not opt for bionic boobs. I know some of you are thinking that, and I am surprised, frankly, because I already told you I was not having reconstruction. But I know it's hard not to go there. So I'll let it slide this time. I can't give you any more details or I'd have to kill you, of course. Either that, or it would just be TMI.

But the good news was that the cancer had *not*, apparently, spread to my lymph nodes.

At this point, Dr. Stahl received a standing ovation from my crowd.

During the operation, she had intercepted and interrogated the five lymph nodes most likely to have been infiltrated by the damn spots, which she had successfully outed in the first Recon Surveillance and Target Acquisition Op, or RSTA as we spy types call it.

She said we would have to wait for the pathology report to confirm her findings, but that she believed we had gotten ahead of the cancer, and therefore we were on top of it. In other words: mission accomplished, return to base.

From what I understand, my peeps clapped louder than thunder and drowned out the rain at this news.

Chapter 13
Drunkard's Prayer

And by drunkard, I mean to give the microphone here to Dave (while I take a little break to pour another glass of wine) because he's the one who got stuck with a handful of *in sickness* and *for worse* chips. If I were to write a six-word memoir, it would be *Sorry I Cashed "In Sickness" Chips*. And the sequel would be, *I Hope It's "For Better" Now*. Anyway, without further ado . . . Dave.

Joules (or as I call her, Joule, for short, which I prefer to spell Jewel, if you don't mind) is a sucker for Shakespeare. I am a sucker for my Jewel. A + B = C. It's simple math, really. I believe even she could figure that one out and with one hand tied behind her back. Even if it's the one with that little finger she's got me wrapped around.

All that to say, I like Shakespeare too. Once I stood up on a bench in the middle of Borders and recited Sonnet 116 to her—it's one of our favorites of his sonnets. And it goes, something like this… ahem:

Sonnet 116
By Will

Let me not to the marriage of true minds
Admit impediments. Love is not love
Which alters when it alteration finds,
Or bends with the remover to remove:
O, no! it is an ever-fixed mark
That looks on tempests and is never shaken;
It is the star to every wandering bark,
Whose worth's unknown, although his height be taken.
Love's not Time's fool, though rosy lips and cheeks
Within his bending sickle's compass come;
Love alters not with his brief hours and weeks,
But bears it out even to the edge of doom.
If this be error and upon me proved,
I never writ, nor no man ever loved.

Shakespeare wrote, "Love is not love which alters when it alteration finds." Surely he had not considered "the remover" to be a breast surgeon, nor "Time's sickle" to be a scalpel, nor the compass of Time's sickle to encompass his love's breasts.

We're not talking wrinkles, gray hair, and a little extra weight here. This is serious alteration. But when it came down to them or her, clearly they had to go.

I admit, initially I told myself that this will be a good thing. There will be reconstruction. My wife will be perky in her old age. But looking into the details, it quickly became obvious that this was not an option either of us wanted. But I have found, in true love, that there is a *breastliness* that transcends the physical and is more tangible than the flesh.

The only real difference this alteration has brought is that when we embrace, our hearts are that much closer together.

"Love is not love which alters when it alteration finds." As I gaze on her even now, I hear my heart say, "Well then, Will, this must be love."

Chapter 14
Honey, I'm Home

And boy, did I have a hard day.

You might be thinking it was definitely five o'clock when we walked in the door after my mastectomy, and that I was more than ready for my honey to pour me a cold one. And by cold one, I know what you're thinking, but what I meant was an icepack for my chest. Honestly, there was only one thing on my mind during the drive home from the hospital and it wasn't can I have a beer to cry in. The crying would come later. My pain meds hadn't worn off quite yet.

No, what I had was an insatiable thirst, or, a bionic desire, rather, for my own bed.

Unfortunately our minivan is not bionic like me. Yukon may be caffeinated in both name and color, but I would have to describe the ride home as disappointing as decaf—not the rush I needed. It almost felt as if we were traveling sideways and might not ever make it home. But that might have just been the pain meds; I can't really say for certain. Anyway, the drive home from the hospital took *forever with a day trip to infinity,* IMHO.

I don't remember (I blame the pain meds) but I doubt I was a pleasant passenger on this particular drive home (let's chalk that one up to pain meds as well).

In fact, I was probably so "not a pleasant passenger" that my poor hubby was most likely secretly wishing there was some kind of *in silence* vow amendment or something. That's how not pleasant I imagine I possibly might have been.

I was, understandably, drained, physically, from the surgery. But I also had three literal drains sticking out of my chest where my breasts used to be. I felt like a tipsy mutant octopus with three left tentacles spewing forth from whence the damn spots were excised. At the end of each flailing tube dangled a suction bulb thingy, which is where my patience, for one thing, leaked out. And that which didn't drip freely, was, quite frankly, sucked out. It was a little like when you suction a newborn baby's boogers with one of those blue bulb syringe thingies, only baby boogers aren't as nasty.

Now . . . if you are doing the math and scratching your head or thinking you just caught me in a typo . . . I'm sorry, and I think that's really very silly of you, but the third drain was for the lymph nodes that had been taken out.

My tennis girlfriends had brought me a pair of pink pajamas with pockets in the front, so I could hide the nasty suction bulbs inside the pockets. Otherwise I would've had to safety pin them to the front of whatever shirt I put on, like some gross accessory or gothic bling.

I wore my pajamas home from the hospital—that's how dressed and ready for my bed, sweet bed I was.

I had all my sheep in a row and was ready to commence counting. But I wasn't the only one in a hurry to crawl under the covers and chase *Z*'s. Everyone in our sloooow-moooving vehicle was so exhausted that it's good that there wasn't a carbon monoxide detector in Yukon, or it might have driven us crazy beeping all the way home. Anyway, all that exhaust made us even more driven to get home.

Dave was so tired I don't know how he managed it all—or me, for that matter. But I've watched *Monk*, so I think I'm qualified to say "Here's what happened."

Dave has superpower sleeping abilities in the literal "blink of his eyes" sense. What I mean by that is, I'm pretty positive he actually switches into deeper REM gears each time he blinks. I have proof. For instance, once, when he was reading a bedtime story to the kids, he fell asleep in the middle of a sentence. There we were, barely hanging on to the edge of our seats waiting for the dénouement; there he was "taking five." Another time, he snuck in a little power nap while making a left turn into our neighborhood. If you're thinking that maybe I'm just a boring driver or something, let me clarify that it was *Dave*, in fact, who fell asleep during his own boring left turn.

I think it's fair to say that after my mastectomy I was in one of my high maintenance phases. I also think it's fair to say that Dave tried to do too much. Besides worrying about me like crazy and waiting on me hand and foot 24/7, which he did remarkably well, he also tried to wear the hat of my personal trainer.

That hat didn't fit. At all. I tried to overlook it, since he was tired and all, but he did get snippy with me when he was "coaching" me through the exercises Dr. Stahl had given me to rehab my arms after the surgery. It was true what I'd heard about not being able to move them above my head after my mastectomy. The left side, where the damn spots were, and where the lymph nodes had been removed, was especially painful. Both arms were weak and sore. My ribs felt like I had been in a barroom brawl. I could only sleep on my back. I was glad I had thought ahead and gotten a "just add water and just drip dry" haircut. I wondered if I would ever be able to raise my arms to steering wheel level, or how in the world I would ever raise my hand to hail a taxi or thumb a ride, or how I would go places—whenever I felt like going places again. Even getting dressed was an exercise that sometimes required a little help. If my tennis girlfriends hadn't taken me out on a pre-surgical-special-ops-shopping-mission to buy shirts that buttoned down enough for me to step into and pull up, I probably would have just worn the same old shirt until I could raise my arms enough again to someday hopefully change it.

Speaking of raising my arms above my head, Dr. Stahl had given me some arm lifting exercises to do. This is where I think Dave tried to take on too much and got a wee bit snippy with me—just because I didn't lift them as high as the stupid exercise diagram paper instructed. I think I was probably only a degree or two off, but you know how heated it gets when we quibble over degrees.

It was hard to complain (though, I somehow managed a little) when he was making my recovery such a smooth operation in practically every other respect. He even had the US Open piped into our sunroom, where I spent much of my recovery rooting for the Serbians because I connected with their underdog stories and their dogged spirits.

One of the less than glamorous, if not thankless, jobs Dave had was that of squeezing the tubes into the suction bulbs and then emptying them. I had a hard time liking him very much whenever he had to do this. It really did suck. Literally. And it did hurt a little—I'm not going to lie. Eight days that week those drains sucked. And I had to carry them around in the pockets of my pajamas.

It was an utterly (note I did not try to *moove* you to laughter by milking the obvious elephant in the room by replacing the two *t*'s in *utterly* with *d*'s) draining experience.

Forget peas and IVs. I *hated* those drains. I know *hate* is a strong word, but I had bionic feelings about those drains. If they weren't attached, I'd have totally ripped them out, thrown them down, and stomped them into the ground.

I counted the days till my post-op checkup and glorious removal of those inglorious you-know-whats, like I had crazy math skills. The much anticipated appointment with my breast surgeon was scheduled for five o'clock on a Friday.

That's right, five o'clock. Talk about TGIF.

Chapter 15
Waiting on the Sun

Friday took its own sweet time.

Thankfully my sunroom is a spy, of sorts, like me. Besides its obvious "cover," my sunroom also doubled as a waiting room. I spent the recovery from my mastectomy in this waiting room. Waiting on the pathology report. Waiting to get those damn drains out. Luckily it was a waiting room with a view of the woods out back, and I could see the tennis courts through the trees.

Meanwhile, Matt and Mikeyy dealt with my cancer with one of the most beautiful random acts of kindness I have ever known: they made a path for me from the waiting room to the tennis courts. The most beautiful bridge over troubled waters I've ever seen—laid down by brothers sowing love, sweat, tears, and hope in the dirt. It was like a path to recovery that I couldn't wait to walk on.

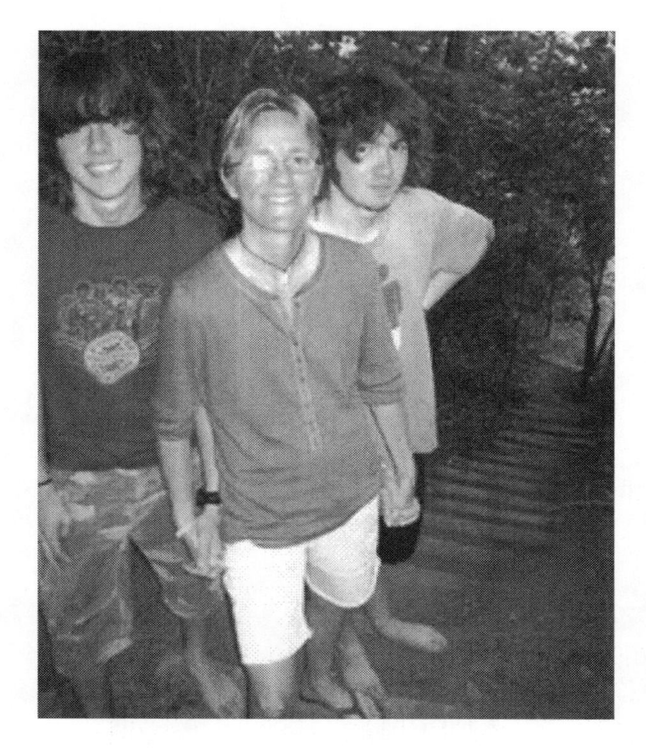

Before the path, taking "the shortcut" to the tennis courts meant slip-sliding down the hill and trying not to channel George of the Jungle. Crawling uphill was especially difficult, and most likely entertaining, after cocktails on the courts.

Up the hill in my waiting room, Dave had "wired" the place (with cable) so the waiting room could also double (triple?) as a press box for my own coverage of the US Open. After all, it would hardly have passed for a real waiting room without cable TV in it.

Besides my running commentary, the main thing on my mind after my mastectomy, if I'm being completely honest, was that I actually, quite naively, thought I would have the surgery, write off a couple of weeks for recovery, then go another six or seven before I'd fully regain my fitness and be back out on the courts, competing with the interclub team I had formed that fall. I was the team captain and I planned to lead my team on the courts, not from the bench.

It didn't quite work out that way.

I don't know if you've ever noticed this, but Evian spelled backwards is *naive.* Being into hydration the way I am and quite particular about the means by which I quench my thirst, I often treat myself with a cold one, and say "Cheers!" to my car when I fill him up at the gas station. I drive a silver Mini Cooper named Rocinante (after Don Quixote's horse) and our tilting at windmills is fueled on his champagne taste in gas. He has this little highbrow *cough-cough* he does whenever someone slips him cheap gas. Like he's choking to death or something. So I have to buy him the best.

I usually pop in the little mini-mart and pop open an Evian for myself whenever I fill him up, because I don't like him to drink alone.

Even though I know what it spells backwards. It's practically the Dom Pérignon of bottled water, if you ask me, and all I'm saying is, I just can't help it if Rocinante comes by his champagne tastes honestly.

Anyway, I couldn't even lift my arms all the way up to the steering wheel during the first few weeks after my mastectomy, let alone shift gears.

But though I might have been idling away in my sunroom, I was definitely revving my engine. I considered myself to be "in training," at least in my mind, as I watched tennis and tried to trick my muscles into memorizing the techniques of my favorite players.

I had my head wrapped around being in neutral. I was OK with this being like a yield sign. I hadn't grasped the possibility that it might be a stop sign, or that I might be stalled.

I was waiting in my sunroom for a *really important* phone call from Dr. Stahl about the biopsy results.

Thankfully, her name is just a homophone, because waiting for the phone to ring to hear whether cancer has spread to your lymph nodes and gone global already feels like the opposite of time flying.

Monday was Labor Day. (Growing up, I had a friend who was born on Labor Day. That made sense. Ever since, I've wondered who was sleeping on the job when they let the word *labor* slide for the naming of a day off. I wish somebody would pay me to name things. For instance, OPI nail polish colors: Wine Me, Dine Me; We'll Always Have Paris; and Romeo and Juliet. How much fun would that job be? And, if you look up those colors, does it really surprise you that they are all wine colors?) As I was saying, Dr. Stahl had already told us not to think she was stalling if we didn't hear from her until Tuesday, since it was a holiday weekend.

Her office did call on Tuesday—late Tuesday afternoon—to let us know that the pathologist's office wasn't stalling either, but that there was a backlog due to the holiday weekend. We would have to wait another day. I had previously relegated my racing thoughts to the back seat of my mind. At this point, I had to buckle them in good.

Nobody said anything about the last time we had gotten a phone call from Dr. Stahl.

The last time we had hoped for good news. The impact of the bad news we got last time did give me whiplash. But my hope survived. Shaken, definitely. Who wouldn't be a little bruised after hearing the *C* word? But not stirred. From my earlier spy-ops training, during my case study of James Bond, I'd learned that shaking stirs up the consistency, while stirring just wrecks the flavor. Bruises the gin or something. Which sounds rather violent, if you ask me. Which is why I don't even own a swizzle stick any more. Besides, the thought of drinking a bruise is just gross. Unless, I guess, you're a vampire. Anyway, I admit that I'm a picky eater. I don't like peas and I do like a little sweet mixed in with the bitter. But shaken, not stirred. Definitely not stirred.

This time I was braced a bit, waiting for the phone call, but still hoping for good news up ahead.

Dr. Stahl called my house on Wednesday, September 3, 2008, with the happy report that the cancer had not spread to the lymph nodes!

The biopsy showed that the left breast still had cancer cells, as Dr. Stahl had suspected. (Good riddance hot boob that tried to kill me!) There were also some benign lumps on the right breast, though they were not malignant. (Wolves in sheep's clothing, if you ask me.) Dr. Stahl said the mastectomy left plenty of good margins and she believed, therefore, that she'd gotten all the cancer. We'd still have to do complete scans to verify that it hadn't sneaked anywhere else. The finding that it hadn't spread to the lymph nodes was not just good news. It was the best news we could hope for.

I'm not even kidding when I tell you that when she called, it was five o'clock in Cincinnati.

Can you get a hangover from good news?

Next on tap was TGIFriday. Time to lose the drains and begin wrapping up loose ends.

I changed into the gown Dr. Stahl's nurse, Rita, handed me, and parked myself on the examining table. Rita came into the room and engaged me in a healthy dose of idle chatter as she lifted the lid on my gown to examine the two tubes on the left side.

Voilà! I think my eyeballs nearly popped out of their sockets in shock at how much it actually hurt when she extracted those tubes. Either that, or the tubes were somehow connected to the muscles that held my eyeballs, and they practically catapulted my eyeballs across the room when Rita yanked the tubes out. I wasn't feeling nearly as chatty as she stealthily dodged my feet on her way to dislodge the tube on the other side.

It only took about two minutes for Rita to extract all three tubes. And by extract, I mean ouch! It's the same principle as ripping off Band-Aids. Only worse. Way worse than childbirth worse. At least with childbirth, you get a cuddly baby out of the deal, which has quite the amnesic effect. Bloody bulb triplets, not so much.

Now don't go getting the wrong idea about Rita. I don't want her to be deluged with nasty letters, because she is, after all, still my nurse and I am still under her power, I mean care. Anyway, *normally* she has pretty decent bedside manner. When she's not ripping out, I mean *extracting* drain tubes. It's just that extracting tubes sucks, as much as the tubes suck.

So, after pulling what felt like yards and yards of spiraling garden hose out of my chest (if you've seen the movie *Alien*, you know just which scene I'm talking about), the tubes were out! Just like the damn spots. Most likely they are all rotting together in a biohazard heap somewhere. Which is fine by me. I know that sounds like misplaced aggression, but if you only knew how satisfying it felt to say that, you might even feel like throwing a few rotten tomatoes at those damn drains with me.

And after a glass of pinot grigio on my back deck the second we got home (it was definitely sometime after five o'clock), I noticed that my pain and nerves were becoming more manageable. I think that much of the pain after my double mastectomy was caused by the pressure of the maze of tubes and the soreness in my left underarm where the lymph nodes had been removed. The actual sites of the surgical incisions were not really much of a bother, except for the fact that they made me look like something out of *Frankenstein*.

I also gained a bit of mobility, with no more toting around of the trio of tubes and their accessories. Not to mention some comfort, sleeping without that ever-present fear of waking up in a pickle of a pretzel—which is a great happy hour snack. But who wants to sleep all tangled up in one?

My happy hour, that night, came in going to watch my Redheads perform at an open mic night.

Waiting for the sun. To rise. Not set.

And I'm just taking my time.

Chapter 16
The Oncolo-*gist* or, "Burn and Shine" Time

"Early stage breast cancer diagnosis, excellent prognosis."

I thought this was a lovely prologue to our relationship. In one fell happy swoop, the newest supporting cast member in my troupe, Dr. Elyse Lower, starring as my fabulous oncologist, set the tone for the upcoming act as soon as I entered the stage of her office.

"Early stage breast cancer diagnosis, excellent prognosis."

Dr. Lower repeated her opening line. I decided that it was one of the nicest things anybody had ever said to me. Really, she had me at excellent.

"Early stage breast cancer diagnosis, excellent prognosis."

"Memorize it," she said. And she told me to practice it until I was in character and acted like I believed it. Until I could practically say it backwards. In my sleep. Or something like that. She was pretty serious about me not getting stage fright and forgetting my line. I connected with her confident coaching technique.

"This is going to be your new mantra," she told me over and over and over again, like she was trying to cast some kind of a spell on me that I just felt like falling under. I can't remember if she actually waved her hand and used the Force on me, like Yoda, or not. All I know was that I decided to throw myself into this role, rather than merely being thrust into it, or having it thrust upon me.

"Early stage breast cancer diagnosis, excellent prognosis."

By early stage, Dr. Lower further unmasked my antagonist and staged my cancer. She went over my pathology report, step by step with me.

My cancer's stage name was T1N0Mx.

Stage left: the T stands for the size of the tumor. Mine was caught miraculously early, for being a high-grade (3) aggressive cancer, and Her2 positive to boot.

Center stage: the N stands for the lymph node involvement. Mine had zero, zilch, nada, none, as Dr. Stahl had previously said (and did) "Cut!" right on cue, which meant curtains for my cancer. (Boo cancer! *Throws another rotten tomato at it*)

On another "aside" note, when I asked Dr. Stahl how much "weight" I'd lost with the double mastectomy, I was delighted to find it was almost Shakespearean in scope, as in just a wee bit Shylock of a pound of flesh.[24]

Stage right: the M stands for whether the cancer had spread to other organs. Mine had the unknown variable of *x* by it because we wouldn't know until we did a series of scans from head to toe. More pictures. I tried to keep my feet on the ground and not let all this media attention go to my head, because the last thing I felt like having was a big fat head. Especially since it was about to be all bald and shiny like a cue ball in the next act. We went ahead and penciled in a zero, with hopes of tracing over it with a Sharpie, after all the scans.

Gotta love Sharpies.

Besides the bright lights of the bone and CT scans, I also had a MUGA scan, which assesses the heart to make sure it's healthy enough to take the chemo. It's also used to establish a baseline since the chemo I would be on sometimes messes with the way the heart pumps.

Besides all those photo shoots, I also did a couple of interviews with people researching my backstory. Dr. Lower had referred me to a genetic counselor for genetic testing. Another freaking test I couldn't study for that I was nervous as hell to pass. I was hoping and praying big-time that I didn't have mutant genes that my teenagers would have to worry about inheriting from me.

If you've read this far into my story, you are probably thinking, like I was, that just growing up as my understudies is enough for anyone to have to deal with in life and would result in years of counseling. Not to mention provide plenty of material for their own memoirs, which will probably be best sellers. And I'm not just saying that because I'm their dearest mommy.

But seriously, I needed to pass this test.

Dr. Lower also set the scene for the fade-in to the chemo cocktail part of my story. Cancer is a pretty hard act to follow as far as antagonists are concerned, but my chemo cocktail was waiting in the wings to make its debut as the next vile villain trying to take down this leading lady.

The scenario was that I was to have twenty-four rounds of chemo.

I hoped they had some pretty big boxing gloves in the prop box.

The playbill for my chemo cocktail read as follows: first on tap was the Adriamycin/Cytoxan mix, every two weeks for a total of four rounds. This was followed by a Taxol/Herceptin chaser, every three weeks for a total of four rounds. And I would down Herceptin cocktails, or Hercep-tinis, as I preferred to think about them, every three weeks, until I had belted down a year's worth of them.

Twenty-four rounds of chemo: 1-2-3-4-5-6-7-8-9-10-11-12-13-14-15-16-17-18-19-20-21-22-23-24. That was like two-dozen eggs' worth of chemo cocktails spilled all over my calendar.

It was T minus burn and shine time. Talk about a refining fire. I found myself bookended by two of the biggest inciting incidents in my life: cancer and chemo.

It was going to be a veeeeeeerrrrrrry looooooooooooooooooong year and a half.

The other side of chemo seemed so far away that it might as well have been at the other end of an ellipsis. I couldn't see that far.

All I could see was cancer chasing me, and me chasing it with chemo cocktails.

I stopped thinking about the future.

I did doubt. About me in the future tense. I did not have conflict within myself or with God about this. I hoped to make it to the future, but it wasn't anywhere on my horizon. I knew we weren't anywhere near there yet, so asking, "Are we there yet?" every five minutes would be wasting time and energy. I needed to "go green" and conserve energy if I was going to make it to see the greener grass on the other side of chemo.

My future was out of my hands. (Like it's ever in our hands. But this was one of those rubber-meets-the-road moments for me. It shook me. To my core.) I could've started counting down my days then. I think that would have been understandable, because cancer is a bitch.

It just is what it is . . . *but* . . . or rather *and* . . . God is good. One doesn't necessarily negate the other. Cancer *is* a bitch and God *is* good. They are both true, at the same time. And part two of that previous sentence is the only comfort I know in the midst of part one.

I thought about making a bucket list. I even wrote *Bucket List* across the top of one of the pages in my pink cancer journal. But I never filled it out. Not that I think there's anything wrong with bucket lists, but in a pretty ingenious twist of my plot, I had an idea that appeared out of nowhere, like a lightbulb hovering over my head. (It was obviously not a halo.) I know this might sound crazy, but I feel like God kind of whispered to me, and told me to count up my days by counting my blessings, instead of counting down my days by checking off my bucket list. A subtle but oh-so-cool trick. It also felt a whole lot less rushed and I hate feeling rushed. I sort of have my own time zone and I sort of don't mind it except for when people get impatient with me. Then it gets on my nerves because I hate wearing out people's patience like entering the Joules Zone sometimes does.

I couldn't grasp the future, but I could seize each day. Break a leg doing it, even. Shoot for the moon, ya know?

We decided to schedule my appearances at the chemo cocktail lounge on Mondays. It seemed best to sandwich it there, between the morning British Literature class I taught and the weekend, which was the intermission I was looking for on the way to remission.

Tuesdays after chemo would be an encore at the chemo cocktail lounge. I would go back to get a white blood cell shot, in my belly, which would prompt the good guy cells to keep up the good fight against any remaining mutant ninja bad guy cells.

Next to be addressed was costume and make-up. I was going to lose my hair. Also, none of my shirts fit me anymore. Wardrobe was going to be a tricky task. I was going to have to "get accessorized" with a port catheter to receive the chemo. This particular piece of bling did not excite me. I actually wavered between doing the chemo by port or IV. To IV or not to IV—that was a question I thought about, a lot.

I was a little nervous about teaching a class of high school students while my hair was falling out—I'm not going to lie. I'm an introvert by nature, and not really an up-front kind of person. I know they always tell you to picture your audience naked, but I've already explained how I feel about nude scenes. And this was a class of high school students, so that would be wrong on so many levels.

So you can see how I felt about standing up at the head of the class—with a naked head.

But the show must go on, so the hair must be written out of my script. For five months.

Even my eyebrows would do a take five. They say timing is everything in comedy. Well, I had recently given in to my daughter's crusade against my un-manicured eyebrows and allowed myself to be subjected to the near scalping sensation of waxing—just a few days before I was diagnosed with breast cancer. They would have manicured themselves and taken their own bow, but that wouldn't have been as funny. It's all about timing, see?

My eyelashes were also going to fade and fall. I hadn't even thought of them as body hair.

Even my nose hairs would take a quick exit. I'd totally overlooked my nose hairs. Who really thinks of nose hairs? I mean, really?

But, yeah, *every* single hair was going to split. And by split, I mean au revoir. As in, I was soon to be as au freaking naturale as a newborn baby's butt. Methinks that's enough said.

The sweetness of the deal was that I would not have to shave my legs or armpits after the literal fallout from downing chemo cocktails. For five months. I don't mean to brag or anything, but it is one of the few "perks" of chemo.

OK, this might be a little TMI, but the truth is, I hadn't actually shaved my armpits since before my mastectomy. My left armpit hurt too badly from the lymph node-ectomy; therefore, my right armpit would have nothing to do with my razor for symmetrical principles. My legs even joined the cause, in solidarity. I appreciated the sentiment, because really, who likes shaving their legs anyway?

And when all that razor stubble (OK, maybe it was more like an overgrown forest, but I think you're just splitting hairs and trying to embarrass me) was going to fall out because of the chemo, I mean, why bother? Why not start the sabbatical from shaving a little early? Go ahead and get into character. Own the role.

My hubby likes to think he is a stand-up comic, and bought me a bag of Tootsie Roll Pops so I could walk around channeling my inner Kojak to feel the part. Sometimes I let him get away with stuff like that because I don't mind getting a free bag of Tootsie Roll Pops now and then. I especially like the chocolate ones.

Dr. Lower wrapped up our first meeting by telling me that I got, and I quote, "all the gold stars" for coming in right away when I felt the lump, and for our aggressive battle plan. She said that many women write off lumps as hormonal, not wanting to make "much ado about nothing." Instead, and unfortunately, many women decide to wait and see if things change after their periods, and sometimes longer.

That's what I almost did.

Thank God I didn't.

With the aggressive and fast-growing nature of the damn spot I found in my left breast, that would have been a "Ya snooze, ya lose" prognosis for me. As in the *big* snooze.

So this is my desperate plea: If you are reading this, please put down the book for a second and go to second base with yourself. Or let the one you love steal second base if you prefer. I'm serious. And you should be serious when it comes to feeling your own hot boobs. But nobody says you have to be so serious that you can't have a little fun with it. Save the ta-tas has created a product called Boob Lube if you'd like to go all out and be all fabulous about it.[25] Heck, pour some champagne while you're at it. If I still had ta-tas to save, you can bet there'd be a bottle in my shower. The cool thing is, just having a bottle of Boob Lube sitting in the shower is a reminder to check. There are even instructions on how to do a proper self-check on the back of the bottle.

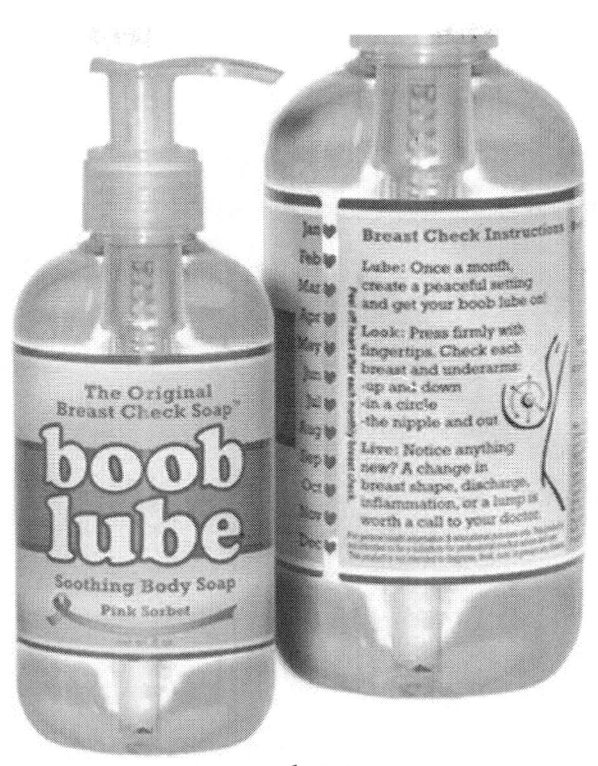

www.savethetatas.com

So go ahead. Shut the book. Just do it. I'll close my eyes. And when you pick up to read again, I'll be waiting here, to finish my story for you when you get back. If you are afraid you'll lose your place, then just dog-ear this page (along the dotted lines at the upper right-hand corner of the page) and then take a pencil and put a little *x* marks the spot at the end of this paragraph so you remember where to pick up reading again. It's important to use a pencil. First of all, pencils are cool. Also, you can erase your marks. That way if you feel like getting felt up again, you can do so at your leisure, and when you're done, it's your secret. Here's where part two of my plea comes in: please do not take any damn spots lightly.

This does not mean I think you should panic if you find a damn spot in your breast. There are lots of "not bad" things a damn spot can be. I've had more friends than I have fingers and toes who have found lumps in their breast since I was diagnosed, who have had them checked and found them to be, thankfully, nothing.

A couple of weeks after my mastectomy, my friend Celina was putting her nine-year-old daughter, Amy, to bed when Amy started crying. Celina asked her what was wrong, and Amy said she was scared she had breast cancer.

"Why would you think that?" Celina whispered over Amy, as she held her close, trying to calm and comfort her.

When the sobs subsided, Amy lifted her nightshirt, and said, "Mom, I have a lump in my breast."

"Sure enough," Celina told me the next day, "there was a little breast bud, starting to form." And sure enough, she and her husband Scott, who just so happens to be a doctor, were able to reassure their sweet baby girl that she was simply on her way to becoming a woman.

Amy was on the verge of her tweens. Her "lump" *was* hormonal. But I take off my hat to her—even if I'm bald. She was self-aware and savvy enough to go ask her doctor, who also happens to be her daddy, about it. You might even say she was a spy like me.

My damn spot began in a duct and had already begun multiplying to three damn spots, spreading outside the duct to the breast when Dr. Stahl stopped it in its tracks, and removed the tracks for good measure. Thank God.

I think he nudged me beyond writing it off, to mentioning it to Dave, who made me go to the doctor the day after I found that damn spot. He orchestrated the speed and manner in which we got past the first Herculean hurdle of breast cancer. So all the gold stars really belong to him, which is appropriate, since he made them anyway. But I do like looking at them, wishing on them, chasing them.

---

[24] Shakespeare's *Merchant of Venice*

[25] http://www.savethetatas.com

Chapter 17
I Run?

September 15, 2008. It had been almost a month since Dr. Stahl had said the *C* word to me. It had been almost two weeks since she had saved my life by cutting into my body and removing the damn spots.

I stood in front of the mirror and scanned my scars. My chest still looked a bit like Frankenstein. But not as bad as when I had the stitches zipping from armpit to armpit. I know the stitches sewed me back together and all, but I felt a whole lot better after Rita, yes, Rita, unstitched me.

I had never had stitches before so I was scared silly that it was going to hurt. It was five o'clock by the time I got to Dr. Stahl's office, but I'd already taken a Valium before I left home—that's how nervous I was about the unstitching.

It was a waste of Valium. I didn't need it. It didn't hurt.

Far from coming unglued, I just counted down the stitches till there were none.

I was so relieved to reach this particular mile marker. (My philosophy is that if you celebrate the small stuff, you have a reason to have a party every day. It's always five o'clock somewhere, you know.)

It was a small step, but it was forward. And I knew that every step I took, no matter how small, left my mastectomy and those damn spots further behind me.

I had my game face on as I dressed in front of the mirror that morning for Cincinnati's 2008 Race for the Cure.

Could it be any clearer where my life was now heading? It was practically written on the mirror. With my mastectomy in the rearview, the damn spots in the dust, chemo up ahead, and the Cure at the finish line, I stared Frankenstein down and got ready for the race.

On my marks. Exactly.

Get Ready. I took a really deep breath before I attempted my first "impossible thing before breakfast"[26] that morning: to raise my hands above my head in order to put on my pink survivor T-shirt.

I secretly wondered if I even technically counted as a survivor . . . yet . . . since chemo was the next leg of my race, and I hadn't exactly survived that yet.

I was such a newbie.

But I had a pink shirt to put on, and it said SURVIVOR on it—in all caps.

I was a survivor. I am a survivor.

I rubbed down my scars with Vitamin E cream and suited up.

Get Set. My friend Celina had set up Team Evanshire for me sometime around my bra burning. I went into "training" right after my mastectomy. At first I was lucky to make it down my street to the cul-de-sac and back. Also, lucky for me, was the fact that Celina's house was on my route. Her front porch was my halfway mark. It was also my very own oasis.

Celina lives seven houses down, or about seven hundred feet. So yeah, most of my training was rather rigorous short-distance intervals.

Exactly a week before the race, I threw my glove down, in the ring, along with my hat, and did two miles. It was a very leisurely, and obviously un-timed, two miles.

The day before the race, I decided to throw down another two miles. This time we clocked it.

Fifty minutes.

Twenty-five-minute miles.

I was a bit out of shape since my college volleyball days when I used to run a 5:50 mile, but I tried to cut myself some slack since I just had my hot boobs cut off. Which I thought would make me more aerodynamic. But then again, like I said, I'm not very good at math.

I wasn't really sure if I could actually make the whole 5K, but I was set to give it a go.

Go. So I totally Veni, Vidi, Vici'd it.

No. I didn't exactly win, or, for that matter, even technically run the race. But I finished it.

I have no idea how I did it, except for the grace of God, and a little help from my friends.

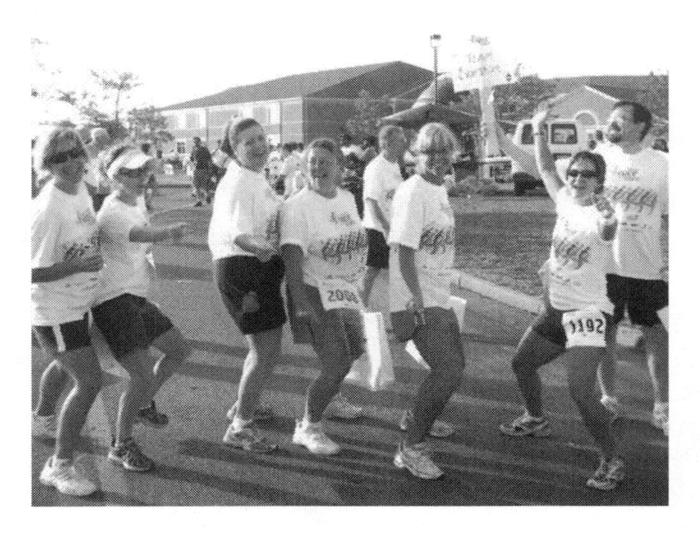

There was another survivor I'd seen at the start of the race who moved me as I began walking. Now *she* was a survivor. To me, *she* embodied racing for a cure. I didn't even try to keep up with her. But I followed her, even if I was super slow at first. Everybody has to walk before they can run. Just like my new superhero, Heather Ray, did years ago when cancer took her leg. But that didn't stop her, and there she was, walking all over cancer and blazing a trail. How could I not make it to the finish line with someone like that leading me?

A funny thing happened on my way to the finish line, though. By the time I *finally* made it to the finish line, it had run out of hot air and deflated.

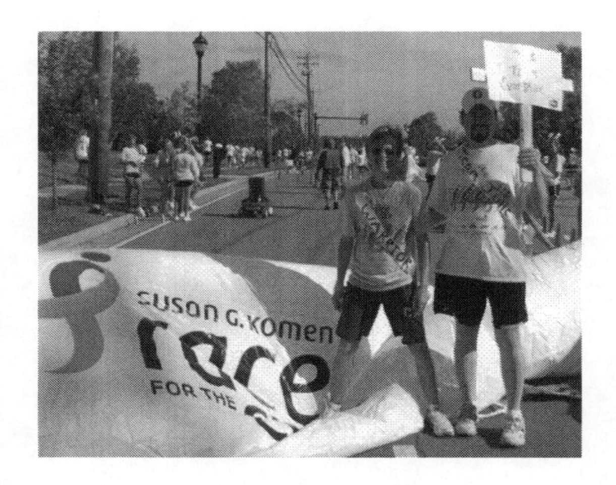

So I stood on it like I was the one who had taken it down.

I walked right over it.

I walked for hope. I walked to feel. I walked for the truth. For all that is real. (And yes, I was channeling me some Melissa Etheridge.)

I walked, flanked by my friends and family, who walked with me and for me. That's about as real as it gets. That's true love. I definitely felt the love that day.

I made eye contact with hope.

I walked for life and for the Cure.

I walked in memory of Sue.

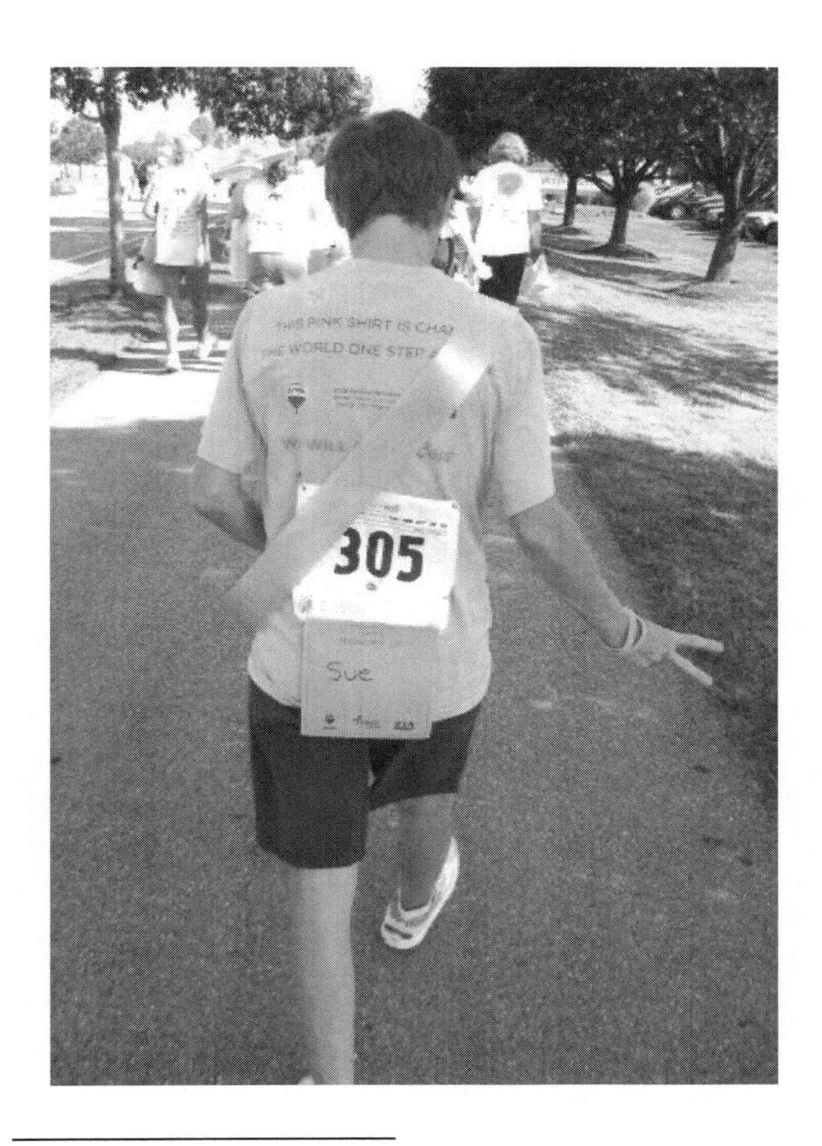

[26] *Alice in Wonderland*

Chapter 18
Come Sail Away

When Dr. Lower scheduled me for a "port," I imagined that somebody with a twirly mustache, shiny cuff links, and a silky white tea towel draped over his perfectly poised left forearm, was going to bring me a glass of wine—and maybe a plate of bleu cheese—as an aperitif, to take the edge off my chemo cocktail. Boy, was I wrong.

We had the impression that the port surgery would be a piece of cake after the doublemastectomylymphnodeectomynottomention drainagetuberemovalontopofthelumpectomy. I like to have my cake and eat it too as much as the next foodie but *Ace of Cakes* did not leave fingerprints on my piece of cake. More like army bootprints.

Having a port catheter inserted usually isn't a big deal.

But haven't we already learned that *usually* usually doesn't apply to me?

The point of the surgery was to dock the port catheter in my vena cava, where it would act as an express route for my chemo cocktail, bypassing the twenty-four IVs, and in so doing, sparing me at least twenty-four stabs.

I initially stressed out about the port because I was worried that it would get in the way of my tennis. I realize that sounds ridiculous, but I was still trying to wrap my brain around how to fit cancer into my life and frankly, it was being a pain in my ass.

But then again, I don't heart IVs. At all. So it was pretty much a no brainer that I was going to get the port. I just had to dock my brain on the idea.

"Easy as pie," they said.

So I took a bite.

It bit back.

Dave thinks I had such a hard time with the port surgery just because I'm, well, petite.

Petite, my syrah.

I think it most likely had to do with the Herculean task of cutting through my tennis pecs in order to find the sweet spot into my vena cava.

That, or it might've, could've had something to do with the accumulation of five weeks of surgeries and procedures having taken their toll.

The day started off badly, and way too early. It was five o'clock when I had to wake up to get ready for the hospital, but the bar was closed.

And, of course, I couldn't even have a freaking cup of coffee.

I didn't exactly hop into Yukon feeling like I was on top of my game for more pokes and prods (even if it meant I would be spared at least twenty-four further IVs) let alone another surgery.

I had just spent the whole weekend wishing things would slow down so I could catch my breath, so I'd feel like I was going into the chemo phase a little more prepared, rested, stronger. Feeling a little more like myself. But I knew that wasn't a luxury I could afford.

I didn't want to leave regrets that my Redheads would have to live with.

One of the most fun, but also genuinely helpful sayings that I've come across in dealing with cancer (then chemo, and every curveball since) is, "It is what it is." The port had to dock in my vena cava if I was going to sail away from cancer. My course was set. There was no choice and there was no time to waste: it is what it is. It kind of reminds me of the theme song from *The Doris Day Show*, from back in the day when I was a kid, the old days when you actually had to get up off the couch and walk across the room to change the channel. (I know, right?!) Anyway, I used to imagine myself sliding down the banister of that twirly staircase. Now that I'm grown up, I imagine myself surfing down that banister. So que se-freaking-ra sera, cancer. It is what it is.

Matt drove to the hospital.

Dave and I were both way too exhausted and on (almost over the) edge. We spent the drive arguing over whether Matt should hug the centerline (my way) or the right line (Dave's way). My theory is that the oncoming cars will move but the mailboxes won't. Dave had recently proven my point, which I made sure to point out, just to be helpful.

He said the mailbox had it coming.

Anyway, he tried to explain to Matt that the arguing was our strategy for training him to drive under pressure, but Matt saw right through him on that one.

I had homeschooled him, after all.

Things went from bad to worse when the nurse had trouble with my IV and couldn't seem to chase down a vein. But oh, how she tried. And oh, ouch, the bruises she left up and down my arm before finally tracking one down in my hand. If you haven't seen my hands, they sort of look like iguana hands. Not super attractive, but good veins that make me wonder why they don't just start with those hulked-out ones instead of digging around my scrawny arms.

That poor pre-op nurse was stuck with me for a while, as she then encountered difficulties in drawing blood for the CBC test. Something about my blood flowing "as slow as molasses" is how she put it. Her day obviously didn't start out any better than mine.

But I could feel her needle up to my elbow.

It did drive home the point that the port was the way to go.

I was actually relieved to get out of pre-op and into the OR after the IV to end IVs. I was almost happy to be wheeled away, even if it was into the OR. After a quick joke, complete with port wine reference for the operating crew, the kind anesthesiologist cast a happier spell over the IV, and the next thing I knew I was waking up post-op.

The port was docked. I was good to go for chemo. Not excited about it, but ready. No more IVs for a good long time.

Once we got home we all crashed hard. So hard, in fact, that we all slept through my scheduled dose of pain meds. Until . . . I woke up shocked by the pain. And, unfortunately, we'd forgotten to stop off at the pharmacy on our way home to fill the prescription for my pain meds.

BIG mistake.

When I woke up crying, Dave was already at the pharmacy getting my pain meds, but my poor Redheads didn't know what to do with me, in pain like that. I may be only five-foot-three, but my threshold for pain is at least twice my height, and there I was, with the pain lapping me. I was not coping very well, at all.

Yeah, I'm a control freak, I know. But especially when it comes to pain management. I do not recommend *ever* getting behind the pain. It's a long hard road catching up with it, once you fall behind. It's like a detour where you keep ending up where you started. Or like a quick trip going nowhere in Yukon.

The Redheads hit the panic button and called Dave, to "help him hurry."

Of course he *was* in Yukon, but he did eventually make it home to help manage me, I mean, to help me manage my pain.

We spent the rest of that day chasing the pain and trying to lap it and get ahead of it once again. Dave set his cell phone to go off every four hours to keep us from snoozing anywhere near the margin of error. We didn't want to let that ever happen, ever again. Never. Ever.

I spent the following day having a hard time dealing with the side effects from the pain meds. At some point I found myself wondering if the extreme nausea and dizziness I was experiencing was more of a problem than the actual pain. The doctor switched my pain meds and voilà—it was time for a little R&R. Finally. It seems that, for some reason, I can handle Percocet via IV but not via pill. Seems it trips over my gag reflex and leaves a bad taste in its wake, which puts the gagging on loop.

Thankfully, that problem was a piece of cake to solve. Which was both convenient and in good taste. Which paired well with my birthday the following day.

Chapter 19
Better Days and Birthdays

If September 2008 was a sandwich, I'd have to say that, for me, the bread sucked.

The bottom of the sandwich was definitely the butt end to end all bottoms of a loaf of bread: my mastectomy. "A totally enriched? pasty, white flour heel of a piece of bread that gums up like glue in your intestines experience," is how I'd phrase it if I were writing a review. I would so totally not order it again.

But as everyone knows, a sandwich must have a platform to build on, so if your bread sucks like mine did, it's time to get creative in the kitchen.

So yeah, it's like I dipped in the breadbox, snagged a bag, untied the twist tie, and reached in and grabbed . . . two flimsy heels matted together. That's the bread I had to work with. I could've said *daggonit*, and decided not to make a sandwich after all, having completely lost my appetite, and I think that would have been perfectly understandable. My mastectomy sucked *that* bad.

But I was hungry.

Mostly I was hungry to keep being my kids' mum. To finish my job of homeschooling them. To do a good job at it. To follow them following after their dreams, and into their lives. To see what their adult lives look like. To cry at their weddings. To dote on their future children.

My grandchildren.

I really wanted to see what life after homeschooling looks like. What was I going to be when I finally grew up?

Would I make it there?

I wanted to grow old with my hubby. Or at least be able to prove that yes, I will still love him when we're sixty-four.[27]

Twenty years down and I still had twenty-two to go.

I was hungry for time.

The beginning of September didn't seem like the best start to all that.

The end of September, and my sandwich, my chemo cocktail, looked just like the butt bread on the bottom. Honestly I wasn't looking forward to biting into that one. I was terrified of chemo. But, every butt has two buns, so instead of saying *daggonit*, I made a Dagwood of it.

The bread, even if it sucks, is still a potential carrier of good things inside.

And like I said, I was hungry, so I decided to pile on everything and the kitchen sink, to see what crazy concoction I'd come up with, and basically make the most of it. It would be the entrée before I could have my dessert: time.

What else was there to do?

Thus began the stacking and condimenting of my September sandwich.

The first layer was the good news that Dr. Stahl had gotten good margins on the damn spots.

The second was finding that the cancer had not apparently spread to the lymph nodes.

That's a pretty good beginning, no matter how badly your bread sucks.

The third layer was the MUGA scan report, which said that my heart was healthy, functioning normally, and good to go for chemotherapy. It was cool watching my heart beat, but I couldn't help but wonder why in the world my heart wasn't heart-shaped, because somebody was flashing their poetic license in that name game. Speaking of, I also tried to figure out, if I were a Brach's candy heart writer what would I write on my heart?

The fourth layer was a triple-decker CT scan (chest, abdomen, pelvis) report, which came back with no signs of cancer! This was the beginning of the non-literal weights being lifted off my chest (as we have already previously covered the literal ones that were *literally* lifted) and Dave's as well (though his were entirely non-literal). He had been wound pretty tight through the initial sandwich-making. Sometimes I wondered if September was, in some ways, harder on him than on me, since I had spent much of it under anesthesia or on pain meds. Dave had no pain meds. Which didn't seem quite fair. And it's not like I shared.

The fifth layer of this hero sub was the bone scan report, which also came back with no signs of cancer!

The sixth layer was the port. The port was like someone topping my sandwich with sautéed mushrooms, like they were doing me some kind of a favor. It's just that I have textural issues with mushrooms. Mushrooms, peas, and ports.

All the poking and prodding to date had not been for naught, because from head to toe, it appeared that I was cancer-free! Which is exactly what we asked God for at the prayer meeting when we began our battle. He heard our prayers and it seemed good to him to answer them by raining down mercy on me. There I was, swimming in mercy and feeling like splashing!

Up to that point, I'd been feeling a lot like the Will Ferrell character in *Stranger than Fiction* who kept a tally to see if his story was going to end up being a comedy or a tragedy. I know that my ultimate story will eventually have a happy ending, cancer or not, because this life is not really the end of it all . . . but even this story within my story has the comedy side way tipping the scales.

How could I not thank God, the author of the happy ending I believe is somewhere down the road?

So we thought it only appropriate to sandwich the occasion with another prayer meeting, this time with the happy theme of praise to God, for healing me.

Coincidentally, the praise meeting fell smack dab on my birthday, whereas the prayer meeting fell on Dave's.

Coincidences crack me up.

And that's what I call the Dagwood to end all Dagwoods.

Even if the bread sucks.

And yes, there was a side dish of pink ribbon cookies that Amanda and Kiley made over at Kiley's house on the day of the prayer meeting. It must've taken longer than expected, tying all those pink ribbons in the dough, because Amanda ended up getting a speeding ticket rushing home in time for the prayer meeting—where she was leading music with her band. Wasn't funny then. Is a tiny bit now.

She got her license suspended for ninety days, but with limited privileges of being able to drive to college, beauty school, work, and to take me to chemo. I wasn't able to make it to her court date, since I was in the hospital having my MUGA scan. This grieved my mommy's heart not to be there, more than I can say. But I can't even imagine how Dave felt having to juggle the two of us that September day.

All in all, I'd have to give him a thumbs-up.

As for my September sandwich, it was like an initiation into the cancer club—a communion of sorts. Because I downed mine with a glass of pinot noir.

In other words, it was five o'clock. And I said, "Bottoms up!"

---

[27] "When I'm Sixty-four" by the Beatles

Part II – A Chemo Cocktail

Round 1
Everyday Is a Winding Road

It didn't occur to me that it might have been slightly ambitious to consider my first round of chemo cocktails as the halfway mark of my breast cancer journey.

I realize that from the time I found the damn spot, to spot removal, I'd only torn seventeen leaves off the calendar. That wasn't even enough to get me out of the longest month of my life up to that particular fork in the road. The leaves outside were still green too. Some things are clearer in the rearview mirror. *Everything* seems clearer once the chemo fog lifts.

But back then, just removing the hazard of the damn spots felt like half the battle. I tried to psych myself up and think of it as the hardest part, since it could have been the end of the road if I hadn't cleared that milestone.

Although September was a big orange blur from the bumpy ride of recovery after having my breasts cut off, not to mention the falling leaves, it was a clear sign that I had made it through the summer heat, safe and relatively sound.

Despite the fact that I was still facing a fifteen-month long and winding road of chemotherapy, I was hoping to give August a chance to make it up to me the following year. And the next. And the . . . well, it was going to take quite a lot of really awesome Indian summers to make up for the one of 2008. But I'm the kind of girl who likes to give people and months a second chance. When I think of my own second chance, it humbles me and makes me feel like I just might be the luckiest girl in the whole world. How could I not pay that forward?

Even though getting a port two days before my birthday and starting chemo two days after seemed a lame way to catapult off a second chance at forty-three years old—it was my route (to) forty-four.

There I stood, staring down twenty-four rounds of chemo cocktails, which felt a little like straining at the gate before running like a chicken with its head cut off through the narrow streets of Pamplona, with all those bulls nipping at the heels—and me running in *bright red running shoes* . . . still.

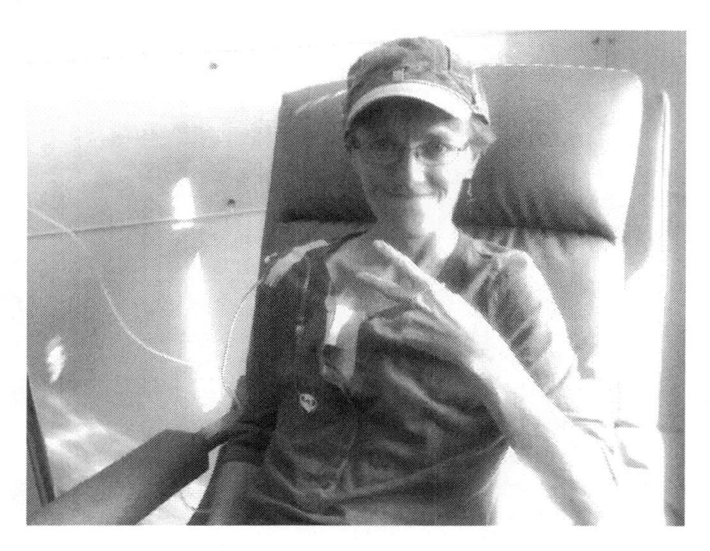

This is where I channeled my inner Hercules. Now I know Hercules had only twelve terrible labors, but the gods were against him, making him do the terrible things that led to his terrible labors. It seems the gods really must be crazy, and surely they drive us all a little crazy sometimes. But thank God there is redemption.

I know I was facing double the trouble of Hercules, but for some reason I don't pretend to understand, God seems to be for me. I have no idea why he is so gracious to me. I know he causes the sun to rise and the rain to fall on both the good and the bad.[28] It's not like I think I'm good or anything, but even though I don't generally get up early enough to see the sun rise, it is usually right outside my kitchen window after I wake up smelling the coffee. Regardless, the sunshine makes me happy whenever I do rise and see it shining. It makes me grateful to be an object of his affection.

That is pretty much the gear I shifted into, on the way to downing my first chemo cocktail.

I was very much on edge about it. How does one prepare oneself for poison, which is the only antidote we have right now for something much, much worse?

On top of the fact that I didn't really feel "up" for chemotherapy. Four days before my first chemo cocktail, I had surgery to implant the port catheter into my vena cava. A month before that, I had surgery to remove both my breasts, and five lymph nodes. Two weeks before that, I had surgery to remove the damn spots. I was feeling like a wreck. All I wanted was to pull over at a rest stop. I just wanted to catch my breath. Unfortunately, due to the aggressive nature of the cancer, catching my breath would have to come later. But the good thing about *later*, is, that it's always something to look forward to. Something good to plug into your factory-installed GPS.

There was no time for a rest stop, but we did manage to fit in a pit stop the night before my first chemo cocktail. Inquiring minds want to know what kind of a last supper a soon-to-be-chemo-patient-with-taste-buds-under-construction feasts on before famishing. Well, I started off with a coffee martini. The clock stops at five o'clock the night before your first chemo. Then I ordered fish and chips (we were at a favorite local Irish pub, The Brazenhead, breaking the fish and loaves with good friends) and a Blue Moon with an orange wedge. Of course I had dessert: crème brûlée and an espresso, chased with a shot of Baileys. I figured the grease from the fish and chips lubed me up like greased lightning. And it's always a good idea to top off the fluids before a journey.

The morning after, I took a Valium, discoursed on Dickens and discussed "the best of times and the worst of times" with my Brit Lit class, then went to chemo. It was. All so very. Fitting.

The actual chemo treatment turned out *not* to be the end of the world. My nerves, going in, were duking it out to see who would be the last one standing, even on Valium. The main thing I was worried about was the nurses pressing around or on the port, which was still smarting from the surgery. I was super not looking forward to the first poke into it.

The poke was simply a poke, and an unexpected piece of cake, though I wouldn't go so far as to say it was yummy. Still, it was a quick dose of immediate gratification that I'd gotten the port. Instead of twenty-four IVs.

All I really remember from that first chemo cocktail was that my oncologist's nurse told me she was cutting me off of coffee and wine while on chemo. This. Stressed. Me. Out. Despite the Valium, and the Ativan, and the Benadryl, and the Percocet, not to mention the intoxicating chemo that entered my port.

I'll admit it. Hi. My name is Joules, and . . . I'm a coffeeholic. Even thinking about decaf gives me a headache. Plus, I don't really see the point of it. I mean, I don't want to be a hater and judge others for their views on caffeination—even if it doesn't make sense to me, at all, period, end of sentence.

Coffee is my alpha beverage. The way my hubby tricks me into getting out of bed every day is by holding a coffee cup just under my nose and waving the aroma toward me, oh so carefully, so as not to accidentally get tangled in the slobber running down the side of my cheek. Then he sets the coffee cup on my nightstand. Just out of my reach. I know it sounds cruel, but I don't want anybody to all of a sudden turn on him. Besides this one tiny little glitch, he's a pretty good guy.

Consequently, red wine is the omega beverage I enjoy sipping with my supper. Now, some days I mix it up a bit and have a shot of espresso after dinner. Occasionally, I will have a glass of pinot grigio with my lunch—I'm not a legalist or anything. It's just a rough guide to my life, where there is always the precarious balancing of the stimulants and depressants. But now, it appeared that chemo was going to knock that off kilter, besides knocking me on my keister.

Time sort of stood still when she told me no more coffee or wine. Either that, or the drip-drip-drip of my chemo cocktail took over the tick-tock, tick-tock of the clock, and I lost track of the now, what-was-I-talking-about? Oh yeah . . . time. I have no idea how long I sat in that muted mint-minus-the-chocolate-chip-colored recliner. Some drips were for nerves, some were for nausea, and some were the big nasty chemo cocktail of Adriamycin and Cytoxan. Adriamycin is called the "red devil" because of its color, which maintains its integrity "round trip." In other words, it's normal to see red—pee, when you're under the influence of the red devil. Cytoxan is a derivative of mustard gas. Yes, fighting cancer is full-out chemical warfare.

I had never thought of toxic pee before. Not exactly the superhero power I was hoping for. Nevertheless, I would now be implementing a "flush twice" policy on chemo weeks. "With great power comes great responsibility." I know. Now under normal circumstances, flushing twice is, um, embarrassing. Under my particular circumstances, it bought me my own bathroom at home. An unexpected perk. Even with the gigantic Mr. Yuk sticker I imagined my silly Redheads would put on the door. The bathroom would be mine. All mine.

I don't remember the ride home, how I ended upstairs in my own bed, or if I stopped to use my bathroom. I guess I drank myself under the table with my chemo cocktail. The only thing to do was to sleep it off. I soaked two pillows and two sets of PJs waking up in sweats followed by chills. Followed by sweats . . . ad nauseum, but thankfully, not followed by ad hurlium.

I had thirty hours' worth of anti-nausea meds that Dave arranged in a pill dispenser, made a spreadsheet, and set his alarm for, which became our chemo week regimen. They left me in a stupor, for which I'm grateful, since that first chemo week remains fuzzy in my memory.

Tuesday was pretty much the same, except I had to go back to my oncologist's office for a white blood cell shot. I was nervous as hell to get it because of the achy side effects associated with it. I found myself getting quite jumpy anytime anyone came near me. I felt a little bit like yelling, "Everybody stop touching me!"

I was, however, worked up over nothing. Nurse Lisa gave me the shot in the belly, which sort of distracted me, since I'd never had one there before. And it was really no sweat at all. Except for all the sweat I sweated worrying about it beforehand.

Besides the nausea (though the anti-nausea meds *did* keep me from tossing my cookies, they *didn't* settle things down enough for me to actually eat any cookies), I had a headache from hell that I couldn't seem to shake. I blamed it on the coffee rations. One a day was not enough.

By Wednesday I was a little less loopy, and getting antsy to stop feeling so crappy. In a desperate move, I talked Matt into driving me to get a forty dollar haircut that might not see me through the week. At the time, I felt it was of utmost necessity, since my bangs were in my eyes, and it did seem to be one thing over which I actually had some control. With Matt's help, of course.

Can I just say that my boys were amazing the way they took care of me during the worst of times of chemo weeks? I was so grateful to be homeschooling, because it was such a gift to have my boys there with me. Even though they were shouldering things I wish they didn't have to.

I know it had to have been a huge relief to Dave, who had somehow, so far, kept all the plates spinning. I don't think a guy has ever tried harder—in the history of the world. It reminds me of Lucie Manette's devotion to her husband, Charles Darnay, in *A Tale of Two Cities*, which I was reading with my Brit Lit class. Dickens penned, "She was truest to [her vows] in the season of trial." Darnay was imprisoned in a tower in Paris during the French Revolution. Lucie would go and stand in a certain spot for two hours every day, where she could not see him, but that he might catch a glimpse of her, just so he would know she was there for him. That pretty much describes how it was for me in my season of trial.

By Thursday I was trying, very hard, to be able to tell everyone who asked me that I was turning the corner and feeling better. I was able to eat a bit more, and even took a very brief walk down the cul-de-sac. But the headache wore me down till Friday, when it finally lifted, a bit after the fifth day of only one cup of coffee.

Then on Friday night my Mini Cooper broke down on Dave on his way home from work. I didn't have a mini breakdown, but I thought about it.

Saturday was a better day. Every day I was getting a little bit closer to feeling fine.

I turned the corner on Sunday. It was a good day. I went to church. I had a massage with a therapist Dr. Stahl had recommended. I went to LensCrafters with Dave to help him pick out new glasses. Then I took a nap. Afterward, Dave and I took a walk. I spent the rest of the evening preparing for my Brit Lit class. Until I passed out, happily spent.

The nice thing about Monday was that it was the beginning of a not-a-chemo week. This is what is more commonly referred to as a good week during chemo—when you don't actually have to go to chemo. I affectionately nicknamed it TGINACW (thank God it's not a chemo week).

The other thing about Monday was that my head started tingling. My oncologist had forewarned me that it was a sure sign that my hair was ready to fall like the leaves were falling. I wrote a sonnet about it, to mark the occasion of my forty-third birthday:

Sonnet Number 43

It's always been a curious thing to me
That the trees bare themselves before the big chill;
Seems a tree needs its leaves for a midwinter dream.
Truth is, I'm not ready for winter. Still

It's coming, like seasons are wont to do.
Last year there were no words, just wonder . . . and
Tennis balls were green; now they are pink, too.
It's a lot for me to comprehend.

There is no complaint, though, in my bones;
I hope I can still say that when it's cold
And I'm bare. All I know, is the one who runs
The weather is the one whose hand I hold.

So comes the winter. So I'll bundle up
With hats and friends. So "Cheers!" as I drink this cup.

[28] Matthew 5:45

Round 2
O Where Is My Hairbrush?

I was nervous going in for my second round of chemotherapy in the same way I was nervous when I went into labor with my second child, Matt. Approximately two seconds after Dave threw my overnight bag into the car, I had second thoughts. And not just because one of his favorite things in the world is speeding to the hospital when I'm in labor—which is enough to put a girl in labor. I don't know if it was the way he revved the engine and said, "Maybe we'll get pulled over this time and get a police escort! Please, can we? Huh, Joules?" All of a sudden I realized I was heading straight for transition.

I practiced my breathing all the way to the hospital.

One of the nice things about holding your first baby for the first time is that you pretty much almost instantly forget about transition.

Until you go into labor again. Then it all comes back. The way the hand on the clock moves way too slow in the middle of a contraction, then mysteriously speeds up in between, while you are trying to rest up for the next one. The chocolate éclair you smell on your hubby's breath that does not help you concentrate. The moment the doctor *finally* says it's OK to push. The second you realize, "Oh crap. I didn't take very good notes on that chapter in *What to Expect When You're Expecting*!"

Flash back. Oh crap. Flash forward. Oh crap. *Rev-rev*. Oh. Crap.

I was not exactly channeling my Little Engine as I desperately tried to remember how to breathe.

"Choo-choo-choo . . . He-he-he . . . Ha-ha-ha? No wait . . . that sounds like Jason from *Friday the 13th*. Oh crap. Now *that's* stuck in my head.

"I think I can, I think I can," I thought. "He he. Ha ha." This Little Engine was chugging away. Up. A. Very. Steep. Hill.

The first chemo'd hit me like The Little Engine's freight-train-carrying big brother. Head on. But the nausea had passed. I had passed the toxic pee. Two weeks had passed. I didn't know if I thought I could, but I did. "Oh crap. Is it already chemo Monday again?"

It was time to get ready to teach my Brit Lit class. When I came downstairs to grab a cup of coffee, Mikeyy noticed that there was hair all over my shirt. I went back upstairs to check my pillow. The pillowcase could have been my shirt's twin. I tossed them both into the laundry chute, carefully pulled a clean-shaven shirt over my head, and went to the head of my class. With hair. One last time.

But first, I downed a Valium with my cold coffee. I was already nervous enough about chemo to make my hair fall out. Plus I was straining extra hard to keep it in until after Tuesday, hoping I wouldn't be bald on Matt's sixteenth birthday.

We continued marching through those worst of times, to better times in *A Tale of Two Cities* in my Brit Lit class. We had tea and biscuits, and then I headed off to chemo.

The oncologist visit took about four hours from start to finish, not including drive time. Dave had taken to calling them mis-treatments. I took a different tactic, calling them my chemo cocktails. Spun either way, name-calling was our survival mechanism. And it cracked us up, which made the medicine go down easier. Cracking up really is the best medicine. Way better than a spoonful of sugar. There ain't no amount of sugar to help the chemo go down. I'm just going to say it: chemo sucks.

Here was the drill: As soon as my class was finished I'd meet Dave at home. I'd rub some lidocaine all around the port area, to start numbing it for the poke and the IV drip. Then I'd cover it with Saran Wrap so it wouldn't make my shirt all gross.

Dr. Lower's office is about a half-hour's drive from the Evanshire.

When I arrived, I checked in at the front desk and filled out a form. It was a little like a multiple-choice test, rating my level of nausea, pain, and et cetera, on a scale from one to ten. I've never been good at multiple-choice tests. I *always* second-guess myself. And don't even get me started on true-false tests. Anyway, thankfully, this was not one of those torturous, true-false tests. Each question was followed with follow-up questions, followed by a fill in the blank.

Do I have any new symptoms to report, questions for the doctor, or do I need more pain meds?

Do I have symptoms? I could write a freaking book.

Do I have questions? How much time do you have?

Do I need more drugs? Is that a rhetorical question?

I so much prefer fill-in-the-blank tests. Give me a blank to fill and I feel a whole lot more confident that I'll eventually find my way to the answer.

After I turned in my clipboard to the grader, I mean, to Rebecca the receptionist, I plopped down in front of the TV outside the lab. I watched a little Food Network while I waited to get called back to the lab to have my vitals checked and to get a blood test, to make sure I was up to snuff for chemo. I made sure they stuck my middle finger so I could flip off the cancer. I know it was silly, and that I was being all passive-aggressive toward the cancer, but the thought of the SpongeBob Band-Aid I was going to get made me feel like a bit of a smartass.

When the blood was being all shy and coagulative, I apologized and gently pointed out that wine is a blood thinner, so I had definitely done my part. I tried not to play the blame game or anything, and Nurse Fatima seemed to take it all in stride. Also she laughed at my joke. Which made me feel freaking hilarious and a little better despite all her finger pricking. Which is pretty good bedside manner, if you ask me.

She gave me a sticker on my lab test result sheet. If that's not proof I handled the situation above and beyond diplomatically, I don't know what is.

Next I watched a little more Food Network while I waited to be called back to see Dr. Lower. She reviewed my blood counts, examined me, and gave me two big thumbs up, in a so-far-so-good kind of way that made me feel like a little bit more of a badass. And then she asked if I had any questions.

I had a little pink notebook with pages and pages of questions. I never trusted myself to remember everything I wanted to talk to Dr. Lower about during the Q&A portion of my visits. Especially since I was usually teetering somewhere in between Valium and the intoxicating chemo cocktail. I needed a script that I had prepared in advance of the nerves, stress, and drugs.

No wonder they call us patients, is what I'm saying.

Anyway, she said I could have a glass of wine with dinner, once I turned the corner from chemo week. That pretty much summed up St. Paul's advice to Timothy for his stomach issues.[29] I was so having stomach issues. The nausea, coupled with the fact that my body was starting to get used to the one lonely cup of coffee a day, made me feel like I was driving one of those old fashioned cars at Kings Island that runs on a track that doubles as a safety guard that won't let the car go off the course. You step on the gas and kind of, sort of, steer, but you can't veer off, even if you wanted to. Which makes it safe even for kids to be in the driver's seat. I loved that ride when I was a kid. I think I thought I was really driving. I was fine with being tricked into thinking I was driving. And everyone knows you shouldn't drink and drive anyway.

After I checked off all my questions and scribbled down all Dr. Lower's answers (which I wrote sloppy, on purpose, since I was quoting a doctor), I headed up to the third floor, to the chemo cocktail lounge.

The first time, a nurse had taken us into one of the private rooms so she could instruct us and walk us through the chemo drill step by step.

This time we went into the common room where a dozen or so of my fellow patients sat in vinyl recliners, hooked up to IVs and doing chemo cocktails. I didn't feel like drinking alone.

I was so anxious when I entered the room that all I was thinking about was the Ativan that I couldn't wait for them to put in my IV. Unfortunately, they were out. The Ativan tap had run dry and I. Needed. Ativan. I threw myself a little pity party. Then I threw a little fit and said, "Figures," and sulked until some of the other drugs finally kicked in. I felt bad about acting like that over Ativan, but sometimes my attitude jumps the track.

When I was little and I'd have a bad day, I'd say, "What a day (sigh)... What (heavy sigh)... a day (tiny, pitiful, whisper of a sigh)."

It was pretty tragic the way I drew it out slowly, inserting sighs in just the right places, and then the repetition, for emphasis. I guess my little outbursts were cuter back then. At least my mum and aunties seem to think so, since they can't seem to get enough of telling that story.

Once I was hooked up to my chemo cocktail, I had some time to sit there in my recliner. I tried to get my mind off my own bratty self by reading the book I'd assigned to my Brit Lit class: *Emma.*

Another brat. How appropriate.

I didn't know if I thought I could do it again. But I did. I downed another chemo cocktail. Now the score was two down, twenty-two to go. Which wasn't my favorite way of thinking about it. I needed a better spin on it so I wouldn't feel so overwhelmed. I needed to think "I can." So I decided the best way was to concentrate, for now, on the flight of the Adriamycin/Cytoxan chemo cocktail. That score was two out of four. That sounded much, much better. That meant I was halfway through the first flight.

Luckily for me, I'd seen *What About Bob?* so I knew the importance of baby steps.

We got home just in time for dinner. In case you're wondering, no, we did not carry on like Bob at the table even though my neighbors, tennis girlfriends, and co-op friends were all taking turns delivering ridiculously amazing meals to the Evanshire every day of every chemo week.

Which was a pretty big change of pace since I love to cook, even if I sometimes seem like I'm channeling the Swedish Chef. One of my favorite times of the day is usually around, you guessed it, five o'clock. It's when I pour myself a glass of red and start frying up the pancetta. If I'm cooking, say Italian, I'll crank up a little Deano, to the tune of "That's Amore" or some kind of mambo music. Then I'll heat up the EVOO, sprinkle in a little rosemary, chop and drop a generous heap of garlic and onions, and watch the family come out of the woodwork. Pavlov rang a bell. I don't need a dinner bell. Just give me garlic and onions.

The funny thing is that nobody in my family likes onions except me. Which normally translates into more for me. Which definitely speaks my love language. But even though they can't resist the alluring scent of sautéed garlic and onions, they look at me like I must surely hate them if they happen to find that I neglected to sift out one tiny sliver of an onion from their marinara sauce. They don't exactly wear lab coats to dinner, or even eat with scalpels, generally, but you'd think the dinner table was a gurney, sometimes, the way they can all dissect a meal just to make sure there are no onions.

Chemo put a major kink in all this fun.

I couldn't exactly manage to chop, drop, and dance around the kitchen as per my usual. Most importantly, it was off-season for my taste buds. The chemo made everything taste like dirty mashed potatoes.

I'm Irish. I dig potatoes, especially with the skins on. Now I have nothing against dirty rice, but I like my mashed potatoes clean, and preferably with garlic. Toss in the nausea and the mouth sores, and throw in an episode of thrush (which I got after my first chemo cocktail) and I had a hard time getting anything past my poor, stunned taste buds, or the hurly burly bouncer that my misfiring gag reflex became.

My chemo diet consisted mainly of bananas, rice, applesauce, and toast. Which makes the thrush make sense if you think about it, since it's a yeast infection babies sometimes get. And if that's not a baby diet, I don't know what is. If that wasn't bad enough, I learned that this is commonly referred to as the BRAT diet. Everybody's a wise guy, even the cancer-diet-acronym-developers, apparently. At least they didn't stop with the applesauce. That would have just been cruel.

Luckily for my family, we had plenty of non-BRAT food gracing the dinner table at the Evanshire during my chemo weeks. Bob would have probably gotten irritating at our table. But we probably wouldn't have said anything. Well, Dave might have accidentally let it slip. Like once, we had a waitress who was wearing a button that said she'd been working at the restaurant for six months, and he couldn't but ask her when she was due. Besides me liking to cook so much, this is another reason we generally eat at home. A lot.

After dinner, Amanda was running her fingers through my hair and, I thought, enjoying herself a little bit too much while watching it fall through her fingers. (She also likes to peel just about anybody's sunburned skin, so it really didn't surprise me. Besides, who doesn't like to have their hair played with?) Anyway, she might as well have been writing on the wall, as far as my hair was concerned.

The next morning, I took a shower and as I gave my hair a bon voyage shampoo, I looked down and noticed there were quite a few handfuls dancing in the rain, clogging the drain. When I dried my hair it flew everywhere. Talk about flyaway hair. I didn't think about it back then, but I wish I would've had a bunch of balloons to stick all over the walls.

It wasn't coming out in clumps or anything. More like a cat shedding. When I wasn't toweling it off or shaking my head, it was still not terribly noticeable, beyond thinning. But, I didn't feel like shedding like a cat, or waiting for a patch of my head to peek through, so I decided to get the upper hand. I asked Dave to shave it off for me.

He shaved my head then he shaved his own.

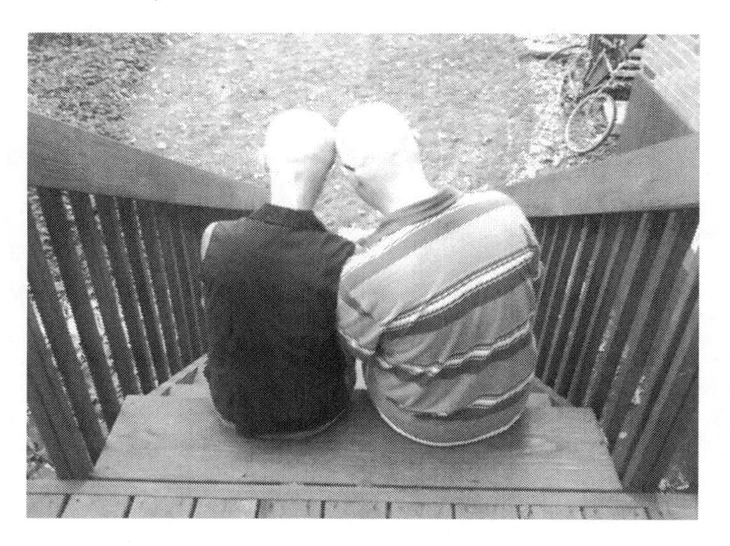

Peek-a-freaking-boo!

First we made a Mohawk and I'm not going to lie—I felt a tiny bit badass. I quickly wrapped myself in a towel to show my Redheads, but they were quicker with their cell phones to snap a picture and post it on Facebook.

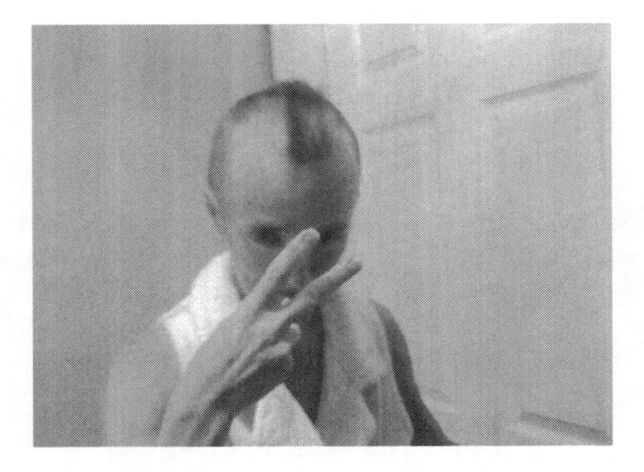

Not exactly the Kodak moment I was going for on Matt's sweet sixteen. But I couldn't have hair and eat Matt's cake too. It was what it was. At times like those, the only thing I know to do is to put on a party hat and grab a fork.

[29] 1 Timothy 5:23

Round 3
Clouds in My Coffee

I've never really thought of myself as a vain person. There are some days when I don't even look at myself in the mirror to see if I have bedhead. If by chance I do catch my reflection in the mirror while brushing my teeth, it's usually before I've had my coffee. In which case I carefully avoid eye contact with that person in my periphery, so as not to be tricked into a pre-caffeinated conversation. It's not that I'm not a morning person, exactly. It's just that I am *quiet* before I've had my coffee. Now give me a glass of wine and I'll be quite chatty. Give me another, and I won't stop telling you how much I love you.

One thing cancer taught me was that I had my own vanity fair going on. I seriously had no idea, until I started having wardrobe issues for the very first time in my life: what to wear with bald? I can't emphasize enough how painfully shy I wasamalwayshavebeen alwayswillbe. Prior to having such a shiny, bald, *bling*-goes-POP, and, did I mention, bald, head to deal with, I dug my role as a behind-the-scenes (or off writing poetry, all by my tortured-artist's-self, wishing for a room of my own) type of girl. What to wear was not really in my vocabulary.

The latter half of my twenties was what I like to refer to as "the diaper bag years." Once I hit thirty-something and retired from changing diapers (can I get a hallelujah?), I hung up my diaper bag. It took me about a month to realize I wasn't forgetting something every time I left the house. I had to re-center my own center of gravity as well. It felt a little like someone had jumped off the other end of the see-saw, after being so used to having a baby on one hip, balanced by a diaper bag, which coincidentally usually weighed as much as the baby. I have no idea why tiny tots think they need to tote about their weight in goldfish crackers, pacifiers, rattles, and an odd assortment of tiny shoes that refuse to stay on their feet, but they do. At least mine did. Which meant that I did all that lugging around of my adorable tots and their ridiculous amounts of totables. And I never thought of it back then when I was young and naïve, but don't pacifiers and rattles cancel each other out? I'd say I felt a little like a pack mule (with a rattle, instead of a cowbell) but I really don't feel like having you think I'm some kind of a jackass—so nix that.

As I was saying, leaving the house without my hair was a little déjà vu-doo-ish to that first month without my diaper bag. Minus the bewilderment, of course, because it was obvious what I was forgetting. Bald is so obvious, it's practically a neon color. Bald is so bright, even Crayola can't touch it and wouldn't put it in the box if it could, because it would just melt the other sixty-three crayons. So you can imagine the crazy pressure involved in dressing up with all that *bling* and POP.

But, if I'm being all vulnerable here, since it's a memoir, and all, the truth is that I was never really all that crazy about my hair. Honestly, I had a really bad double cowlick. That ridiculous cowlick is half the reason I gave up looking in the mirror in the first place, and, basically, trying to do *anything*, at all, with my hair. It was simply pointless trying to make my mop lay any which way but the erratic way it wanted to. Primping has never been my style, anyway. For me, brushing my hair was like making the bed or folding underwear. It was nothing more than a non sequitur, if you will. I do not follow because I don't get the point. The bed is going to get messed up all over again at night. The underwear is just going to get tossed in a drawer, and it's not like anyone will ever know if it has a few wrinkles, anyway. My hair was going to look like a cow licked it. Twice. It was what it was.

Was.

Now, however, it looked like it was five o'clock, the grazing hour, in cow time, on my scalp. I had to come to terms with my bald self, and going out with a hat, knowing that I'm not fooling anybody. Not that I was trying to fool anyone. But I just wasn't in the mood to be a billboard.

It's interesting . . . Before, when I was sick and didn't even know I was sick, I didn't look sick; then, when I was *technically* "better"—boy, did I sure look sick. It's hard to keep straight, especially with chemo brain, which is a for-real thing, by the way, in case you didn't know. For real. Google it. And I'm not just saying that to get you to cut me some slack now and then since I had cancer, and did chemo and stuff. Although if you end up googling it and then feel like sending me a bottle of wine or some chocolate or something to make up for your skepticism, I will totally cut you some slack, because that's just how I roll.

In addition to chemo brain,[30] there was also the initial shock to my system whenever I happened to catch my reflection in a window, or the microwave, as I passed by. I usually ignore mirrors because they are obvious. Except for rearview mirrors. Now they are tricky. But windows, and especially the microwave, sometimes trick me into glancing into the looking glass. It took me awhile to get used to that strange person looking back. I couldn't help but wonder what I looked like to others. I felt like such an incongruity, and a vain one at that.

I didn't feel like just standing there and channeling this narcissism, so I had to get over myself, tune into my inner Elvis, and just leave the freaking building, thank you very much.

It probably doesn't make any sense that one of the first places I debuted my bald head was in the hot tub at my tennis club, the Five Seasons Family Sports Club. Things had thankfully slowed down from the siren pace of part one of my cancer battle and, not to complain, but I was feeling like I might have gotten caught under the wheel of the ambulance and dragged around a bit in the process of having my life saved. I mean, I was grateful, don't get me wrong, but what I really needed was a nice, long soak in a hot tub.

Luckily, all those tennis lessons were about to pay off, because my tennis club had a hot tub.

But first, I had to deal with a pesky little side effect I refer to as *the swimsuit issue*. And by issue, I refer to all that "extra material" now sagging in my swimming suit top. In other words, it had become clear that I had, in fact, become too sexy for my swimsuit. However, it's not like October is exactly swimsuit season in Cincinnati.

Alphabetically swimsuits are next to the snow gear, but not seasonally. I wasn't sure if a pre-alphabet top even existed, let alone one that wouldn't bother my still-sensitive port. It was an almost futile search, but I did finally settle for a pair of underwear and a matching cami from Kohl's. They didn't *exactly* look like undergarments.

The other wardrobe issue I had to deal with was what hat to wear in the pool.

I'm not your typical swim cap type of girl. Seemed a bit redundant. Instead, I ended up wearing my white Nike tennis hat with a black swoosh that matched my intimate apparel, I mean, my one-of-a-kind, anything-but-original swimsuit. I turned my head and looked away whenever I passed a mirror in the locker room. I also avoided looking at my reflection in the pool at all cost, so I was not in the least bit of danger of falling for myself. Even with my sexy unshaven legs.

I almost cried when I dipped my toe in the warm water. Then I splashed right through any reflection, and submerged myself into the hot tub. Every aching muscle sang a chorus of *ahhh*. Even the hair on my unshaven legs seemed to be swaying like reeds to the happy tune.

After I soaked in the hot tub so long my limbs felt like linguine, I grabbed one of those noodle-floatie-things, and jumped into the pool to cool down. Thought I might as well do a few laps, since I was there, dressed for the occasion, and there were lanes, daring me, on my mark, to get set, and go. Challenge accepted. I probably lost a few points for form, if we're being technical, but I did make it four lengths. Swimming backwards, with a purple-noodle-floatie. I tried swimming forwards with one of those kickboards, but I couldn't stretch my arms out in front of me to hold onto it, and when I tried to prop my neck up on it, it I almost drowned. I didn't think Nike would be impressed if they happened to be scouting me while I was drowning. So I kicked the kickboard to the curb. I didn't feel like blowing any future endorsements. Needless to say, I did not attempt the breaststroke (ba-dum-bum).

Come on. You were thinking it.

Besides channeling Michael Phelps, I was also up to walking two miles. If you think about it, throw in a LIVESTRONG bike, and I was practically in training for a triathlon. Which is another reason why I didn't feel like jinxing that Nike deal.

You can't imagine the pep talk I had to give myself the first time I had to teach my Brit Lit class bald. On the very first day of class I'd given my class a heads up, that a short, kind-of-cute, bald chick might be filling in for me in a couple of weeks, and that she would be as badass as she looked . . . so they'd better have kept up with their reading of *Emma*, when she asked them about it.

They are all pretty smart. You have to give them that. The day I walked in without any hair, they were all sitting there like angels. With bandanas on! Such. Sweet. Solidarity. I'll never ever forget that kind gesture. I totally gave them all As for the semester, right then and there. Made my job easier. And it was easy because all I had to do was blame the chemo.

I am teacher; hear me roar. Or see me smirk, really, if you really believe I just gave them As like that. They also had to bring biscuits (and by biscuits, I mean cookies, to go with the tea) to the party, I mean to class, at least one time during the school year, if they wanted to pass my class.

Those were two really big feats, but probably the hardest was the most normal activity: girls' night out. As much as I wanted everything to just be like always and feel normal, it just doesn't feel normal going out with the girls without your hair. Here's the email I sent out in reply to the evite, just to break the ice:

> Joules is in. Looking forward to seeing everyone. Sorry my hair can't make it—except, for the hair on my legs, which I will probably not braid for the occasion, but which I totally could, if I wanted to. So, if you're on the fence whether or not to come, I'll just let you know that it may be the last time you can see my hairy legs until my hair grows back in the spring. Which seems an appropriate time for it to sprout.

It was so good to go out with the girls and do something so normal. I almost forgot that I didn't have hair underneath my hat. But then I could see it in all their eyes: they were dying to rub my head and make a wish. Luckily, we were in a Chinese restaurant that gave out fortune cookies because I think this saved me, and most likely, their delicate tennis-calloused hands, because my head still had razor stubble that could have literally sliced their forehands.

My fortune said, "You will become a great philanthropist in your later years." Of course, the *later years* part made me especially happy. But the philanthropist part sounded just as sweet, since it seemed to imply that I was going to have lots of money to give away, in later years, as in, the future.

I wasn't so vain; the song *was* about me.

Which of course made me think of that Nike deal. I had been following their advice throughout this "hairy" ordeal of going bald: "Just Do It."

So *that's* how I was going to make all that money that I was going to get to give away in my later years.

And *that's* how I was able to walk into my third round of chemo feeling like I was giving an encore appearance at the chemo cocktail lounge: shaken till my hair had fallen out, but not stirred. Channeling my inner Bond girl came through for me in the clutch.

Speaking of clutches, my car broke down. Right after I'd *just* gotten it back from the Mini doctor, who had *just* replaced the clutch. And yes, it was the clutch, *again*. Dave and I were trying to act like a normal couple and go out on a date. We thought it was about freaking time, since we hadn't been able to squeeze in a date since my b.c. (before cancer) days.

We hopped in my Mini and headed downtown to catch a movie. On the way there—I must preface that Dave was doing the driving—we lost fifth gear, then third, then first. In rush hour. Which I thought was odd on a couple of levels. Somehow, Dave managed to get us to the theater on time, toggling between the even gears, and finally pulling an *Italian Job* parallel parking maneuver right in front of the theater. We came, we saw. We were there, after all. And after all, we could stand a little amusement and some popcorn. Logistically speaking, watching a movie would allow for the rush to pass us by so that we could toggle homeward without feeling like we were in a no-win situation playing reality Frogger.

I don't know if it was repair malpractice or—I hate to point fingers—operator error. But Dave blamed the Mini. On the way there he was even talking about how it was probably time to sell R-O-C-I-N-A-N-T-E (like my car can't spell his own name) because I had been struggling at shifting gears. Which was obviously the port's fault. *Not* poor Rocinante's.

What I think happened that evening, was that poor Rocinante got his feelings hurt. He lost his will to go *vroom*. I mean, who could blame him? If there was to be no more chasing of windmills, then what, really, was the point anymore?

In Dave's defense, I don't think destroying Rocinante's spirit was his intention, because he's really not a meanie like that. Even though he likes to think he looks mean with his Mr. T haircut.

One day at co-op, one of my students told me, "You totally look hard-core with that bald head, Mrs. E. You're kind of a badass." I have to admit, that made me feel a little badass. When I told Dave about it later, you could totally tell he really wanted someone to say that to him. However, badass or not, I thought an apology to my poor Rocinante seemed warranted; maybe even a car wash would be a nice gesture.

After the movie we lost reverse and then second in the process of un-parallel parking and trying to get going quick enough to jump to fourth. Unfortunately our route was uphill and that didn't happen. What did happen was that we also lost fourth gear and ended up sitting in the middle of a five-lane street. Downtown. At eleven p.m.

I didn't cry because it was cold sitting on the curb waiting for a tow truck and you know how I feel about icicles on my face. Plus I already looked pitiful enough. I usually make my kids carry around a blanket in their car during the winter and I just kept thinking, "If only I wasn't such a freaking hypocrite." Amanda burst out crying when we walked in the door and told her my Mini broke down. She felt so bad for me that she broke down, too. It was her last straw.

I was tired of straws. Wondered what my last one would be. And it looked as if I'd be in need of that proverbial camel, since my poor Rocinante was back in the shop.

I still hadn't really cried about my cancer. I don't know if that's weird or unhealthy or if it's just me and if that's even OK. I almost did cry when we got that phone call and my kids broke down. But there's something about being a mum and watching your kids break down when they hear you have cancer. Something kicks in when somebody messes with your kids. You're going to kick cancer's ass in a minute, but right now you have to just hold your kids really tight so they know that you're not planning to go anywhere, or do anything but be their mum.

I did shed a few tears one night, all by myself, when the rest of my family went out. I asked if they minded if I stayed home alone to chill, with Chinese and a chick flick. It just so happened that Lifetime was showing a double feature premiere of *Why I Wore Lipstick to My Mastectomy* and *Living Proof*. Un-freaking-canny.

It's funny how I cried more over Geralyn Lucas's cancer than I did my own. Safer to connect with somebody else's story than to break down in the middle of my own, I guess. I didn't wear lipstick to mine, but I did find myself crying over hers, and I was glad that I don't wear mascara. I also connected with her sense of humor, and laughed my ass off, which was just what I needed. It was good medicine.

Living Proof is about breast cancer researcher/superhero Dr. Dennis Slamon, who developed the truly miraculous breast cancer drug Herceptin, which I'd be downing during my second and third flights of chemo cocktails. The movie was such a boost and a primer. It made me so very grateful to him, and I was especially moved by the brave women portrayed in the movie, who went through all the trial phases to help get Herceptin approved to help people like me. Thinking of those courageous and gracious women definitely uncorked a river of tears: happy, healing ones.

When I sat down in my chemo cocktail lounge chair ready to rock and recline Round 3 the next day, I looked around the room like I hadn't looked around it before. One of the things that struck me was that I wasn't the only bald one there. This was my new normal. All these beautiful bald women were my chemo sisters. That was strangely comforting.

When the nurse hooked me up with my chemo cocktail, and before I got too loopy and sleepy, we decided it was time to roll the drum and officially name the port. I figured I was going to be living with the damn thing sitting on my pec muscle for a while, so I might as well have a little fun and give it a name. And now, it was time to choose the lucky name-the-port winner from the contest I'd hosted on my blog. I had a baker's dozen or so to consider. I shook them up, not in a hat or a cocktail shaker, or a lottery ping-pong ball machine thing, but just inside my brain. Of course I didn't stir them. I was just reading them off a list and not literally drawing from literal scraps of paper.

I decided to name my port Rafa, chiefly because Jehovah Rapha is one of the names of God that means the God who heals, and that is where my hope is.

Coincidentally, Rafael Nadal, or Rafa, is one of my favorite tennis players, and his road to number one in the world is such an inspiring story. He's the most tenacious yet gracious fighter in tennis, which is how I hope to fight cancer.

Since I'm a grammar girl, the homophone worked for me.

A close runner-up was Hey Jude. If you check out the lyrics, it's pretty spot on clever. So I decided that it would be the official theme song for my port. Lady Macbeth and Port of Good Hope both got honorable mentions.

All that to say, Round 3 was significantly better than Round 1, and even slightly better than Round 2. There was only one more round in this flight, and the clouds in my coffee seemed to be parting. Which was good, because I take mine black.

[30] http://www.cancer.org/Treatment/TreatmentsandSideEffects/PhysicalSideEffects/ChemotherapyEffects/chemo-brain

Round 4
Hit Me with Your Best Shot

I'm aware that my microscopic stature is not *that* intimidating on the tennis court. But that doesn't stop me from trash-talking with my opponents before a match.

If my team is the home team, one of my first tactics is to spin my tennis racquet to see who gets the serve. I play with a HEAD tennis racquet. On a coin, heads or tails is obvious. But not so, curiously, on a HEAD racquet, making it quite difficult to discern which end is up. But to me it looks like a smile, or a frown, depending on your perspective. So I look my opponent in the eye, and I say, "I've got a happy face, and a sad face. You call it." I know it's cheesy, and I'm OK with that, obviously—a little wine with that cheese? Why yes, please.

Anyway, nobody ever chooses a sad face. But sometimes it lands on the sad face. When it does, I smile, turn around, throw down one of those *mwahahas*, and start serving it up. Love-love. Game on, girlfriends!

If that's not intimidating, I don't know what is.

In tennis, love stinks. When your opponent is about to take her turn serving and she says it's 40-love, it's *not* a term of endearment. You don't want to be stuck in love in tennis. I know it seems to be contrary to *girlfriendology,*[31] but we girls are complex beings, so trust me, love is not the goal when you're playing tennis. Even among girlfriends.

In chemo, love *is* all you need. Chemo doesn't play fair. It schemes to break you—that's its job, to kill the bad cells. But it's so good at its job that it doesn't have time to discriminate between good guy cells and bad guy cells; it just takes them all out, and your hair too.

After my third round of chemo I was feeling like I had three notches in my proverbial lipstick case (since I don't own a real one). Now that I had the drill down, it was time for the trash-talking to begin.

Even if you're microscopic from across the net—*especially* if you're microscopic across the net—you have to be able to trash talk with the big girls if you're going to get anywhere in tennis. And that goes especially for women's interclub competitive tennis. Same thing goes when downing chemo cocktails.

Therefore, once I *thought* I was in the clear from Round 3, I started dancing around like Monty Python's Black Knight, feeling all invincible and stuff.

Yeah, there was the nausea, which felt a lot like morning sickness, that I couldn't do anything about. But I hadn't vomited once so far. And, yeah, there was also the headache that was pretty much the Energizer Bunny of headaches, throughout chemo weeks. I blamed the chemo, which made me feel a microscopic bit better, which was heading in the right direction. By this point I knew it wasn't the caffeine, since I had beaten down my coffee addiction to one a day. It was practically a vitamin, and therefore a weapon in my battle.

"'Tis only a scratch," as the Black Knight would've taunted.

I'd learned to navigate the chemo fog. Having three under my belt felt like a tic-tac-toe. I got all excited and wanted to go ahead and just cross through my *X*'s. But this flight was actually more like the *slightly* more challenging Connect Four. So I had to wait. But I *had* this. Consequently, the anxiety I'd been experiencing from all the unknowns I'd been facing and all the unexpecteds that kept popping up began to lighten up. I was beyond the learning curve. Joules had found her chemo groove.

Life does go on during chemo. Especially when you have three teenagers. My Redheads were my reasons and my priority. Before chemo I multitasked pretty fiercely. During chemo, even on good weeks, I was lucky to do one non-school thing a day. It would generally take all morning to gear up for it, and then I'd need a nap afterward, to gear up for dinner. Then it was bedtime. It just was what it was.

I was psyched how quickly I seemed to turn the corner from Round 3, because I had two, not one, things on the calendar for Friday. Both were in pen.

Friday afternoon was the funeral celebrating the life of Yott's mom. We didn't have the luxury of ever meeting one another following the prayer meeting that had knit us together in my heart. I had prayed for both of the other moms whenever I prayed for myself, so I felt quite connected to them. And now, I felt loss. The boys grew even closer through everything they shared and suffered. Yott drew near to us, and was drawn near and dear to our family.

Friday evening we had tickets for a David Crowder Band concert. Coincidentally, it was Halloween. First came the *trick*: We had ordered the tickets back when we were figuring out the chemo schedule in the beginning, and had miscalculated, thinking it was a not-a-chemo week. Oops. But since it was the *treat* we'd all been dangling in front of us to have something to look forward to, to keep mushing through this chemo groove, I came home from the funeral and rested until it was time to leave for the concert. Then I took a nap in the van on the way there.

The concert was such a treat. Mikeyy lost his voice singing along. Matt got his concert ticket, Amanda and Mikeyy got their Converse, and even I got a T-shirt signed by David Crowder. The front of my T-shirt had the apt title of the album/tour: *Remedy*. On the back of it he wrote, simply, "Mom's Shirt." I liked that. I snapped tons of photos of my kids and their friends with him. Even I got a picture taken with David Crowder. Which was hilarious, given the juxtaposition of his crazy hair and my bald head. My face hurt from smiling. By the end of the night I felt my smile was stuck, like the Joker's.

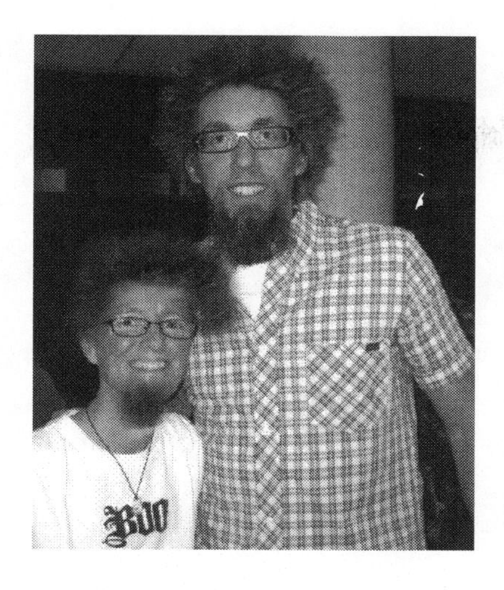

The next morning I quickly realized that I had overestimated myself and done too much. Not that such foreknowledge would have stopped me. When it comes to calendars, pen is pen. I'm normally a pencil kind of girl; I like the flexibility to erase. But sometimes you have to use a pen. On the rare occasion I do, I am not a fan of scribbling it out. Life's messy enough.

The fatigue hit hard. My heart raced every time I got up to refill my water bottle or go to the bathroom, which is a lot of what I spent my time doing. I spent the entire Saturday trying to catch up on Brit Lit reading. I hadn't been able to focus enough to read all that week.

I'd done all my lesson plans in the summer, before I got sick. Otherwise, yikes. I had my students reading thirty to fifty pages a day and writing a two-hundred-fifty-word literary analysis three times a week. In order to lead class discussion on the readings I'd assigned, I actually read along with them myself. I had to. Even if I'd already read the book, I had to re-read so it would be fresh in my mind. I also had to grade and comment on the fifty or so essays I collected each week. On top of that mound of paperwork I had to make time for my own personal research and preparation for class discussion. Overestimate myself much?

So here was my strategy: read a chapter, bathroom break, refill water bottle, and repeat.

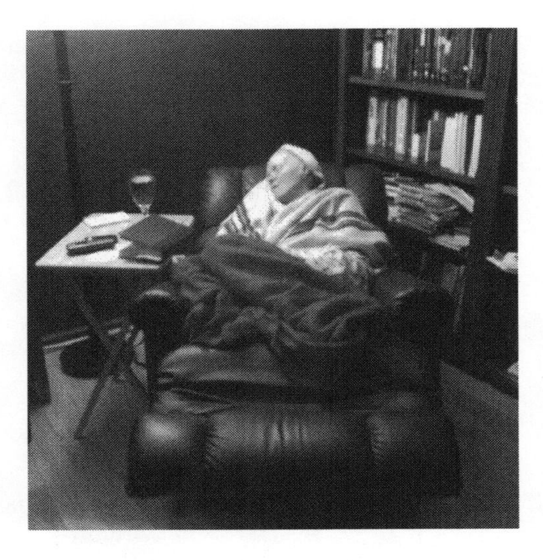

With a few naps, a short walk down the cul-de-sac to fight fatigue and focus my poor chemo brain, plus lots of losing track of what I was doing in between, I did finish. But it was distracting hearing my heartbeat all day. I could hear and time it with the tick-tock on the wall clock. It made me feel like I was racing the clock, since I have a hard time turning off my competitive nature, especially when I can't release it playing tennis. And of course my class was Brit not American Lit, so I couldn't even use the beating heart as a lead-in, teaching Poe.[32] I don't know if racing the clock made me all tense and tight, but my chest began to feel as if things didn't quite fit.

Besides that, the swelling had gone down around Port Rafa and I could feel and see some of the stitches holding the tube in place. This did not help calm down my heart one bit.

The doctor's nurse told Dave that it was usual fare for chemo. It just is what it is. I just had to put my game face on and keep moving toward not-a-chemo week. It took a lot to gear up for chemo weeks, especially as the fatigue accumulated and I began to waste away and look like I felt. I used to carb up for tennis matches; now Dave was trying to fatten me up for chemo. With the nausea and everything tasting like refried beans or mashed potatoes but diluted of all the flavor, it was not an easy job. Finding something, anything, that triggered the salivary glands so the food wouldn't just . . . sit there forever or trip the gag reflex, was not a job I'd wish on anyone. Not even an Iron Chef, like Cat Cora. (There isn't enough Ouzo to subject someone to that. I may or may not be such a fan that I keep a bottle of Ouzo on hand for when she's on *Iron Chef*, so I can down a victory shot with her.) Nevertheless, Dave waited on me, channeling Westley, of *Princess Bride*, "As you wish." Whatever I wished. Often, even though he granted my wish, it wouldn't go down. It got to the point that whenever I actually finished eating something, everyone would clap. And I learned a lot about how small children wrap their parents around their tiny fingers in those attempts to please everyone and make a happy plate.

Not-a-chemo week came, and with it, November. Monday, I taught.

Tuesday I voted. Serendipitously, I ran into my friend Linda at the polls. Linda is a tennis friend and neighbor fighting renal cancer. Doctors removed her kidney after finding two tumors the previous year, one the size of a tennis ball, and the other the size of a golf ball. She was just getting back on the tennis court and was preparing to teach my Mikeyy geometry that year (she was a recently retired math teacher) when she found out the cancer was back in the cavity, her lungs, and breast. She is such a graceful, gritty fighter, like Rafa, whom we both love to watch play tennis. She's an inspiration to me. That she was not only willing to, but desirous of continuing to spend some of her energy (which I am learning is an extremely precious commodity when you are fighting cancer) teaching Mikeyy geometry still humbles me and compels me to pay it forward. I pray for her whenever I pray for myself.

Matt got his license on Wednesday. In other news, my Mini was still broken down, and my computer crashed. C'est la freaking vie. It goes on.

I wrote this poem the night before Round 4:

Some Days I Feel Like Midas, Minus the Gold

'Twas the night before chemo
And all through the house,
My computer wasn't stirring,
Not even the mouse.
Out in the garage
What do I hear?
Nothing, because my Mini
Lost his gears and isn't here.

Despite feeling that way and penning that poem, I still had to teach my class, then put my dukes up, and walk in the chemo lounge. So, like the Black Knight, I was like: "Put up your dukes. Let's get down to it. Fire away." I downed Round 4. And it did fire away.

There wasn't any hiding the cumulative effect the chemo was having on me at this point. I had very little energy, wasn't very steady on my feet, had an even harder time concentrating, and my pulse was racing at 97.

But, unsteady or no, I was back on my feet. "Had enough, eh Adriamycin and Cytoxan?" Because that's game, set, match. I win. Love stinks, don't it?

---

[31] http://girlfriendology.com/

[32] http://www.literature.org/authors/poe-edgar-allan/tell-tale-heart.html

Round 5
Beauty from Pain

They say beauty is in the eye of the beholder. If that's true, then after my first Taxol chemo cocktail, I temporarily lost my grip. I'd say I was channeling my St. John of the Cross and experiencing the dark night of my soul (because it was the deepest despair I have ever known) but St. John of the Cross did not cross my mind, nor was he anywhere near. And honestly, I was in so much physical pain that I didn't really want anyone anywhere near. Which wasn't exactly channeling my inner pilgrim in the Thanksgiving spirit, either.

I'd heard that eighty percent of chemo patients find Taxol to be a walk in the park compared to the red devil. I was looking forward to a walk in the park. I just had no idea that park was on the wrong side of the railroad tracks in Dante's hell.

Was I shocked that I fell in with the twenty percent? No. If you've read this far, then you probably weren't either. If this were a novel, you would *expect* me to throw that kind of a curveball at our hero. But this isn't a novel and I don't make this stuff up. Though it amuses me how fiction is sometimes easier to believe than reality, and how reality can sound so contrived. But I digress.

I couldn't wait to transfer flights from the Adriamycin/Cytoxan chemo cocktail to the Taxol/Herceptin one, mostly to get away from the red devil, but also because I would get an extra good week on this flight. The treatments would be every three weeks, instead of every two.

I felt quite Thanksgiving-y the morning of Round 5, as I applied my own lidocaine and Saran-wrapped Port Rafa all by myself. A few of my tennis girlfriends took me to chemo that day. They'd packed a little pre-Thanksgiving turkey feast for us to gobble as we gabbed. This was the first (and only time) Dave didn't go with me to chemo. And it wasn't easy getting him to stand down and let my girlfriends take me. But this was supposed to be a girls' night out, so I was forced to play the cancer card. I had never used it before, and I didn't want to use it except for emergencies, but I thought the poor guy could use a break.

The one thing about Taxol was that it made me tipsy, which was a not-so-bad start, since chemo always kept me on edge. The dose was equivalent to a glass of wine (on top of the premeds on top of the Valium). Not exactly what I'd have chosen to go with my turkey sandwich, but I didn't feel like complaining since I was in the Thanksgiving spirit.

It was a good girls' night out, even if it was in the middle of a chemo cocktail lounge in the middle of the day.

When the girls brought me home they put me straight to bed to sleep it off.

Tuesday I got my white blood cell shot.

Now, I'd heard about Taxol's side effect of numbness and tingling in the feet and hands. But again, I was concentrating on the percentages, more than on any probability of it actually happening to me. My fingers and toes went numb. I don't think they were shocked, at all, to find I was outside the box on the statistics. In fact, I think they were quite apathetic, actually. Until they realized it meant they would be "cut off" from veggie slicing duty. Then the numbness hit a nerve.

What I hadn't heard about Taxol was that it might make me achy, like the white blood cell shot made me achy. Normally, I could've done the math, figuring that meant achy on top of achy. But I was in a chemo-brain state of mind. And really, it ended up feeling like achy squared, if I were doing an actual audit.

All day Wednesday, my tennis girlfriends dropped by and dropped off side dishes to flank the turkey I was bound and determined to cook with my Amanda.

One of my favorite family traditions is our fabulous famous dancing drunken turkey. The only word to describe it is *yum-O*. Which isn't surprising since I found the recipe in a Rachael Ray magazine.[33] I haven't even *looked* at another turkey recipe since. My poor taste buds were understandably frustrated, knowing I wouldn't quite be able to taste the fabulous famous drunken turkey. But I didn't want that to get in the way of the joy of cooking it. The first time we ever made one was the first time I ever got to host Thanksgiving at the Evanshire. My mother's side of the family all came, and I couldn't have been happier if I'd kept the Sauvignon Blanc-Semillon I'd saved for the turkey all to myself. That turkey was almost as big as Amanda, who, in a bold move that was destined to become our particular twist on the turkey, threw down her apron and picked up the turkey. To show it just who was boss. She took the bird by the wing and danced around the kitchen with it. After she named it, of course. His name was Tom-Tom.

Our third turkey in a row was like tic-tac-toe. We won, even if my taste buds couldn't taste the victory.

The victory was sweet, but shortly afterward, I began to feel like I'd turned a wrong corner and was sliding down a hill. I went upstairs to take a nap to try to sleep it off. But the ache was just settling in for a long dark night of my soul. When it did, I crashed and burned. Hard. And how. I woke up from that nap with my legs aching so badly I thought the pain would suffocate me. By Friday, I was wishing it would go ahead and snuff me out quick. I know that's not the most thankful thing to think the day after Thanksgiving, but it's the awful truth. It was the first time I found myself wondering if I was strong enough to make it through chemo, and to go through it again, three more strikes, I mean, three more times.

There's a line from one of my chemo cocktail songs, "Beauty From Pain," by Superchick that said what I couldn't articulate, better than I could groan. "I know I'm alive, but I feel like I died." And that was pretty much how I felt. I didn't know if I might be dying and I wondered if this was what dying felt like and how long it would take. How much I could take. I didn't think I could make it to tomorrow, and I doubted if the sun would really come out anyway. I was so not channeling Annie.

I don't know how I hung in there to the next day, except for "God's eye is on the sparrow and he watched over me" because frankly, I lost my grip and couldn't hold on anymore. He must have caught me from falling and put me back, because the next day, here I was.

But when I awoke, it was to news that my friend Linda had gone to be with him. We were two ships that passed in the night. She was heading to the light. I would like to have waved goodbye. But it was such a dark night. And then there was mourning.

But there was also symmetry, which I think she'd appreciate, and poetry, which she knew I'd find in her passing as I passed that night. What a shining example she left behind.

When Linda's cancer came back with a vengeance, she didn't check out. She signed up. She aimed big. Linda wanted to go on a mission to Africa to work with a hospice one of her former students, and now, friends, was involved with. But she also did small things with great love[34] that she hoped would change the world.[35] Having recently retired from a long career as a Catholic high school math teacher, when Linda learned that I was looking to hire a geometry teacher for Mikeyy, she offered to teach him. She wouldn't accept any fees. When I pressed, she just said I could pay it forward and make a donation toward Africa and the hospice. She spent herself completely, loving others. Linda gave Mikeyy her "last lecture."[36] She gave him the gift of her time, knowing the price tag on her time. This rocked my world. Changed it. Changed me. She was the inspiration and a significant part of the reason I decided I must continue teaching my English classes through chemo.

Linda had finished her fight and was at peace.

I awoke and was not finished.

It was not really the time for rest. Dave had been having stomach issues that had him doubled over in pain much of the weekend. He thought it was just indigestion, or something that would just "pass." Yet, I did notice that he had been googling *appendicitis* in the wee hours one night. I thought maybe he'd developed a stomach ulcer worrying about me and *everything* else. The guy had a bit of stress on his plate. By Sunday night the kids and I had decided that enough was enough. I was too sick to keep up my end of the *in sickness* bargain to take him, so Matt drove his daddy to a doc-in-the-box, who ended up sending him to the ER. They ran diagnostic tests on him all night long.

It was gallstones. Dave and Matt came home at six in the morning with three prescriptions, a surgery to be scheduled (somewhere in between my chemo cocktails), and a new diet.

Implementing that diet felt like we had reverted to nursery rhyme status and humor. Dave had become Jack Sprat, who could eat no fat. And I was his lean wife, I mean, his wife who could eat no lean because Dr. Lower wanted me to work my weight back up to the triple digits.

Sometimes, from my perspective, I think the world only appears to be nonsensical, like a nursery rhyme, mixed-up and upside down. Sometimes it does seem to be a "very, very... mad world... mad world."[37] But like some wise anonymous soul once said, things are not always what they seem, and it wasn't Mother Goose. I know I go on about "it is what it is" all the time, because, at least for me, it's been helpful to just accept what is, come what may. Complaining about it makes less sense than a nursery rhyme. It doesn't take a wise man to see that it only feeds the madness. The flip side of that coin, though, is that things are not always what they seem. Things might seem to have gone awry, from my perspective, but the truth is, I don't know Jack about perspective, and it's really OK. In other words, there is more than meets my eye. I like to think that even when the world feels upside down, especially then, it's always in God's hands, and somehow, it's right side up to him.

He is the beholder. He made the world and everything, and said it was very good.[38] It is beautiful. It's just that sometimes it's hard to see, from our point of view.

If I hadn't lost my grip, I don't think I would understand that truth as deeply as I do now. Hope slipped through my numb fingers, but it had hold of me. I fell right into his hands, where I was all the time. I can't think of a better place to plant my own perspective.

I wonder what he will do with these ashes? Something beautiful, I hope? No, strike that question mark. Something beautiful. I hope.

---

[33] November 2006

[34] Mother Teresa

[35] Steve Sjogren, Founder of Vineyard Cincinnati

[36] by Randy Pausch. Published by Hyperion, 2008.

[37] By Tears for Fears, 1982. I'm mad about the Adam Lambert version.

[38] Genesis 1:31

Round 6
Breathe

I didn't exactly skip into the chemo cocktail lounge for my second round of Tax-ALL— which is how I decided to spell it since its bite was so bad I needed to amp up my bark. Plus, trash-talking my chemo like that cracked me up. And I can always stand a good laugh, especially whenever I take a seat in my chemo cocktail lounge chair. Like my *Save the ta-tas* T-shirt says, "Laughter heals." I always crack myself up every time I pull it out of the drawer to pull it on. It's a rather compelling PSA. Kind of like Superman and his shirt, only I don't go hiding in phone booths and ripping off my clothes like Clark Kent. I like to layer as much as the next superhero, but I'm not really a suit and tie kind of a supergirl.

I knew it was a passive-aggressive thing for me to do, misspelling my chemo on purpose like that. I know chemo doesn't care if I spell it right or not. That's not the point. I care. Before chemo, spelling used to be one of my lesser-known superpowers. I don't mean to brag, but I did win my class spelling bee twice during my elementary school days. Unfortunately, both times I cracked under the pressure of the bright lights in the school auditorium during the all-school spelling bee. If you were sitting in the audience on those fateful days, you might have thought I had a tick or something, the way I got nervous and tacked an *e* onto *carbon* one year, and then onto *devout* the next. Even though I totally knew how to spell them both. Still doe.

This time, though, I meant to spell Tax-ALL wrong. It had nothing to do with nerves. It had everything to do with control. I'm sure Adam got as much of a kick out of naming the animals as I did when I re-named my newest antagonist: Tax-ALL.

I was fully aware that I was displaying misplaced aggression by doing so. I know that chemo is a pro-, not anti-, agonist. It's cancer's sworn enemy, not my enemy, but—agony is agony. And I've got to be honest since this is a memoir, and by its very nature, nonfiction. Most of the time it sure felt like cancer and chemo were ganging up against me. So yeah, I blamed the chemo. The nice thing about you, dear forgiving reader, is that I know you probably don't even blame me for blaming it on the chemo. So thanks for that.

When something kicks your ass like Tax-ALL kicked mine, once you've coped through the first round, you have to somehow find the courage to walk into the chemo cocktail lounge for three more rounds. And not think of them as three strikes.

Well, it isn't easy. But it's not impossible, either.

Especially if you have a Santa Claus hat and/or some peppermint sticks dipped in dark chocolate at your disposal. Lucky for me, I had both. It was December, so I thought it was time the chemo cocktail lounge began to look like Christmas.

What I didn't want for Christmas was chemo. But I did feel like staying alive a bit longer, so skipping chemo wasn't an option.

I did weigh all the options going in, after my first Tax-ALL hangover.

The way I saw it, the pros were:

1) I had no choice.
2) Once I downed this one, I'd be halfway through the bumpy Tax-ALL flight.
3) The bartender was finally adding the much anticipated Herceptin to this chemo cocktail. Which made me think of Harry Connick, Jr., who had recently starred in *Living Proof*, the Lifetime movie about Herceptin. So with degrees of separation being what they are these days, it was practically like hanging out with Harry. And who doesn't want to hang out with Harry? Or Harry Handsome Connick, as I sometimes call him, when Dave is feeling super secure, since I don't really feel like hurting his feelings.

4) I would have three weeks to shake this round off, and Merry Christmas: no chemo hangover on Christmas.
5) I was kind of getting into the groove of not having to shave.

The alternative and obviously, therefore, the cons, were:

1) Saying "Uncle" to Tax-ALL. The thing is, I don't really like losing.
2) And that's not just me being a sore loser. Losing, in this case, meant giving any remaining cancer cells the chance to get all comfy cozy to the point they might feel like staging another takeover. As in game over.
3) I wasn't in the mood for my own funeral if I could help it.

The pros won out. Except for antics, antidotes, antioxidants (read: dark chocolate), and antipasto, I'm not a very anti- kind of girl. In fact, I rather fall in with the pro-antics types because I like to keep things positive. For instance, even though I'm not a fan of cold temps, I wouldn't classify myself as anti-freeze. Just think what that would do to the ice cream industry. I, for one, don't feel like being classified a hater like that. (Proof: I don't understand why so many people are anti-Monopoly. One of my fondest childhood memories is of playing *Monopoly* with my Uncle Bill, so all those anti-monopolists kind of rain on my parade down memory lane. But not so much that I feel like being all anti-them. That would be like returning evil for evil, and who has time for that?[39] I surely don't have time to waste.)

I've already covered my general distaste for antagonists, but I also have a general impatience for anticipation. I'm not just talking ketchup. Waiting, in general, bores me. Anticlimaxes have the same effect on me. I won't go into antis such as anti-theft and antiviral, because really, nobody likes thieves or viruses. Being antiviral is like preaching to the choir and that is so anticlimactic, it makes me sick.

A little-known fact about me is that I don't do antiperspirants (although it is quite possible that this has become slightly more public knowledge of late). I think I have chemo BO. And yes, I totally blame it on the chemo buzz I'm *still* trying to walk off, because I don't remember stinking before chemo. I think we all agree that chemo stinks, so it just seems kind of obvious. At least this bohemian scent is in keeping with my apparent lack of style—*not* anti-fashion, BTW. It's not that I'm pro-perspirant, but neither am I anti-antiperspirant. And, not for anti-social reasons either. I'm really not anti-social. Just ridiculously, painfully shy. And I think being anti-anti anything is a little absurd, if you want to know the truth. I'm no math genius, but even I know that two negatives make a positive. So really, all this anti-anti business is a little like splitting hairs. And if you'll remember, at this point in my story, I didn't have any, so it's a rather moot point.

Anyway, the reason I don't wear antiperspirant is because when my friend Sue first got breast cancer, the first two things she did were to eliminate antiperspirant and to stop eating chicken breast that had been enhanced with growth hormones. Both of these steps made sense to me.

Many of my survivor sisters have gone through similar mental stress, trying to sort out all the conflicting and ever-changing information out there as to what to eat, what not to eat, what lifestyle changes to make, et cetera. "Wear sunscreen so you won't get skin cancer on top of breast cancer. But wait! Now you are low on vitamin D, which we *now* think may cause breast cancer." Or, "Soy, soy, yay rah soy! Except if you have hormone-positive breast cancer, in which case, boo soy." Or, "Drink red wine. It's good for your heart, especially after all that chemo did its number. But crap, drinking causes cancer." If you only knew how many times I have gotten a link to that article in the email. Seriously, a girl could go crazy trying to sift through all the contradicting information available on the interweb. It's all so—very stressful. And by the way, stress causes cancer.

One thing all the weighing of pros and cons led me to think about was how chemo and Jesus both bring me to my knees. That's the only similarity I can come up with, but it's significant to me. I knew I had no choice but to take the chemo. All I had to do was look at my three kids and there was no question in my mind about that. But give me Jesus, please. I'm not trying to be all religious or anything because I don't really get into religion. Or feel like beating anybody over the head with it. But the truth is, people always ask me about the hope I have because it doesn't seem to make sense in the middle of cancer and chemo. My answer is that except for Jesus, I don't know. It seems legit to mention it here in my memoir. To sign my name on the dotted line, if you will. The truth is, cancer is the enemy here, and Jesus has been more than a friend to me. I'd have to be an ashamed and awfully selfish jerk not to say so. I'm not ashamed, and I don't feel like being selfish, which, by the way, probably causes cancer.

Besides hope and humor, all I know about finding courage is to put one foot in front of the other. Life does go on during chemo. Dave's gall bladder, for example, was not going to wait. We had to find a place on the calendar, somewhere in between my chemo cocktails, where Dave could have the drama queen of a gall bladder removed. Amanda was in the midst of wrapping up her first quarter of college and beauty school for Christmas. Her driver's license wasn't going to be underneath the tree, but she would finally get it back. Matt was dealing with a double ear infection, and Mikeyy had an ear infection and strep. Both were probably worn down from being the most amazing caretakers and companions in chemo history *ever*, while simultaneously being my own personal germaphobe-busters. You can't even imagine the amount of Clorox Wipes and Purell my boys went through, trying to "get my white blood cells' backs." My hunch is that they crossed the streams from the Lysol cans because I didn't even catch a sniffle. Which was good, because I didn't have any nose hairs to catch a drippy nose.

Obviously it wasn't all fun and games in the Evanshire. We were definitely feeling like pomegranate pulp that had come out the butt-end of a juicer. Not exactly what you'd expect to throw in the shaker for a stiff bracer the weekend before the Tax-ALL man cometh.

That Saturday night before chemo was my tennis club's annual Ballers Against Cancer fundraising event. We were partnering with The Tiffany Foundation, an organization founded by the family of Tiffany Floth Romero, in her memory. Tiffany was a fellow tennis lover who fought a long hard battle against inflammatory breast cancer. She was on chemo the last four to five years of her life, without a break. But she fought with honor, on her own terms, and lived and loved to the last.

A bunch of my girlfriends were going, and of course I signed up, too. But inside I was kind of a wreck about going because I was a wreck about Tax-ALL day. Also, I was nervous about being conspicuous at a breast cancer event with my bald head. I told Dave that I hoped there would be other "bald" people there so I wouldn't stick out and be a distraction because it was a fundraiser and it was about Tiffany.

There had been a snowstorm in Cincinnati, which made driving to the event interesting. My kids were waiting on friends they had invited to the event. They were going to follow after as soon as their friends arrived. Then we started getting phone calls telling us that their friends were having a hard time getting to the Evanshire. I pulled the cancer card and told the kids I wanted them to stay home. I was going to be a worse wreck if my kids were out driving on a night like that. I also think part of me was worried that they were having to deal with too much cancer, and thought they could use a break.

When Dave and I walked in the doors at Five Seasons, the first person we ran into, coincidentally, was Tiffany's dad, who told me I reminded him of his Tiffany. I was amazed that I got to meet him right off the bat, and was also shocked that he knew my name. Then I met a girl named Kristi, who used to be bald like me. But yeah, other than that, I was the only bald chick in the building.

Kristi had been traveling down a very similar road as the one I was on. Except, she was only twenty-eight years old, newly married, and recently pregnant when she had been diagnosed, a year before I was diagnosed. Kristi had done the Adriamycin/Cytoxan cocktail while pregnant. She had a healthy baby girl, aptly named Addison Hope, and born, quite appropriately, on Thanksgiving Day, just before she began her Taxol/Herceptin cocktail. Addison was now a one-year-old. And Kristi was about to down her last Herceptin cocktail, just before Christmas. What a road she had traveled. I was humbled, to say the least, by her youth and the incredible circumstances she had overcome, which made my own pale in comparison. And it was obviously encouraging to see someone who had traveled the same road I was on, make it to the other side of breast cancer and chemo. She had been there and done that already. Meeting Kristi was like getting a postcard from hope.

When Kristi got up and shared her story, I was not shocked that The Tiffany Foundation had honored her the previous year. I was stunned, however, and rendered speechless when she, on behalf of The Tiffany Foundation, awarded me a family membership to Five Seasons and free tennis to help me get back out on the courts! I don't know if it was the chemo or what, but I didn't have the slightest clue the evening was headed there.

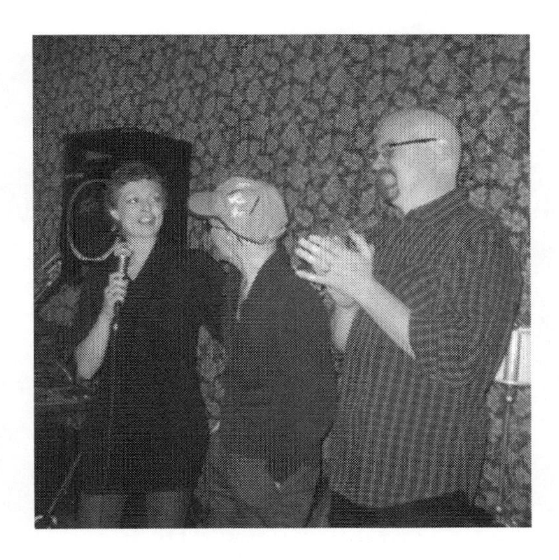

So much for being inconspicuous. What an unexpected boost, and what timing. It's crazy times like that, when I find grace at the bottom of my cup, and the next thing I know I've downed another chemo cocktail and I'm wearing a lampshade, or rather a Santa Claus hat, on my head, singing Christmas carols in the chemo cocktail lounge.

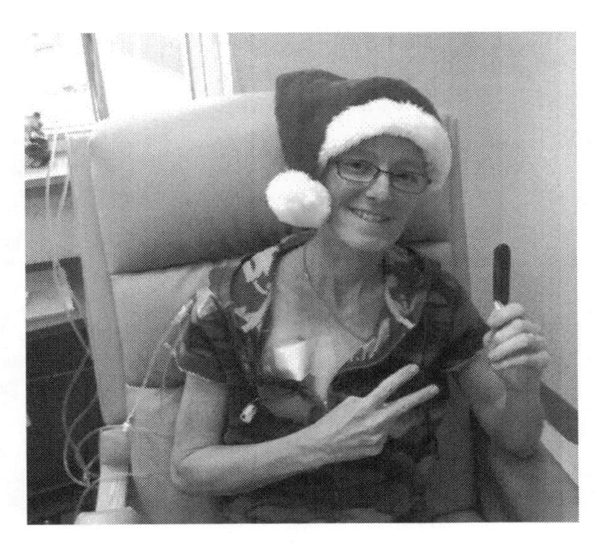

After downing Round 6, I had plenty to sing about. I had one round of Herceptin under my belt. I was halfway through the Tax-ALL. And I had three whole weeks before the next round. It might've been the Santa hat. Either that, or I got tipsy on Tax-ALL, but something put me in the holiday spirit and I found myself remixing a few holiday tunes. And cracking myself up. Laughter, after all, does not cause cancer.

"The Twelve Days of Christmas" is one of my favorite ones anyway, but especially when every day your true love gets you ANYTHING BUT CHEMO!

"I'm Gettin' Nuttin' for Christmas" was not so bad when the nuttin' meant NO CHEMO!

And the famous, "Jingle Bells, CHEMO SMELLS!" Well, that one just feels good to sing out loud.

Speaking of feeling good, I'd called Dr. Stahl's nurse, Rita, to talk to her about Port Rafa, which felt like a Hummer trying to fit into Rocinante's parking space. She told me to call her friend Sharon, a massage therapist, who happens to be a two-time survivor, and now specializes in treating women who've had breast surgery. So during my extra "good week" in between rounds, I completely freaked my body out by having a massage. It was not expecting that at all. For a moment it wondered if it was having an out-of-body experience. What's this? No poison and pain today? Then it remembered pleasure, and at first it was a shock, but then it was just "ahhhhhhhhhhhhhh."

At which point I realized that I probably hadn't relaxed a single muscle nor taken a deep breath since I'd found the damn spot. Sharon told me I was in guard mode, and that it was normal, considering all I'd been through. Her compassion was as therapeutic to me as her skill. It obviously wasn't a deep tissue massage. It was more like a touch of mercy. She kept reminding me to breathe. Honestly, I was holding my breath to keep my eyes from leaking. It was the strangest sensation. I wasn't sobbing or anything, like Mira Sorvino does in the movie *At First Sight.* But I did think of that scene when my eyes were springing little leaks every time she said, "Breathe now."

---

[39] 1 Peter 3:9

Round 7
Dear Santa: I'd Rather Ride in a Limousine

In some ways, Christmas 2008 was like a dream. Mostly a good dream, though, because I didn't want to be hooked up to the chemo tree on Christmas morning, and Santa delivered!

Also, I loved the idea of getting to spend the holidays at the Evanshire.

For twenty years we'd spent most of our holidays traveling to, from, and in between visiting our families in Indiana. Dave and I were both the first to take flight (and clear across the country, to boot) from our families' nests. Coming home for the holidays was, therefore, keeping up our end of the deal for introducing the absence of the hearts-grow-fonder variety. As Dave was wrapping up his electrical engineering degree at IUPUI, he accepted a job offer in Texas and, practically the day after he graduated, we packed up my Ford EXP and I went west with my young man.

We drove straight to Greenville, like we were racing to catch the sun setting where we checked into a Holiday Inn. It served as our home base while we checked out apartments. I threw up when I awoke the morning after we got to Greenville. No, it wasn't a hangover from putting a nightcap on that long drive. Dave ran out and bought the hotel version of a home pregnancy test and we found out I was pregnant with our first child. It was the good kind of pink. Still, this was not exactly the phone call our parents expected to get from us after we'd driven halfway across the country to start a new life there, but there it was. Dave's pretty literal.

We weren't able to travel back to Indy for the holidays that year. I was on bed rest for preeclampsia, and just a couple weeks shy of my due date. Every Christmas after that, though, we took our kids back to our roots so they could soak in the soil. When they were young, especially, this was a priority. We wanted them to be familiar with our families.

About a month before our third child was born, outnumbering us in life and on cross-country travels, we cut fifteen hours off our holiday commute by moving to Cincinnati. When our kids were young, it was relatively easy to attend even everyday occasions with our families. That was before our kids had college, beauty school, work, high school, extra curricular activities, youth group, band, friend and dating commitments, and conflicts with life as we used to know it. Back when we were younger. In my b.c. days.

Cancer changed everything. It did an utterly thorough shakedown of things. All things. Including holidays. I couldn't go to Indy. Chemo had shaken my immune system defenseless. But I was there, alive and kicking in my own home sweet home for the holidays, so that was a good start to something new.

My sister and her family drove in from Charleston, after a detour to Indy to visit our family so they wouldn't be strangers to my toddling nephew Brody. I call him Charlie Brown because he so totally channeled Charlie Brown's head and hairdo when he was a baby. He calls me "Noopy" and it kinda sorta makes me melt.

My dad and stepmother drove over to spend Christmas Eve with us.

My mom drove over for Christmas morning.

Minus the cancer, we experienced a peace that harkened back to the peace on earth and joy that the angels heralded about more than two thousand years ago. There was no Christmas break from cancer, but there was peace in the Evanshire. Maybe it was because of the cancer, or despite it—I don't know—but either way it was a gift.

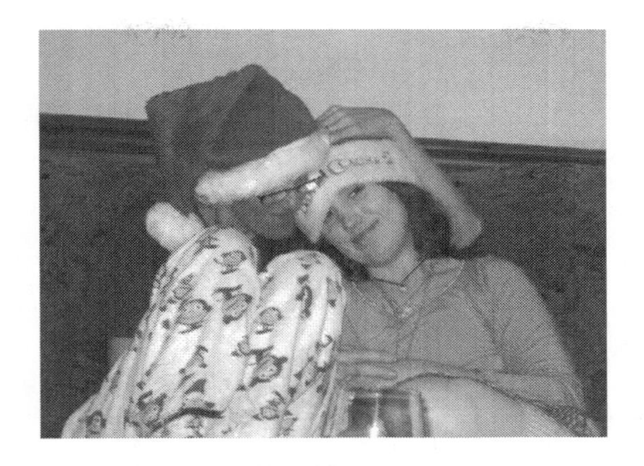

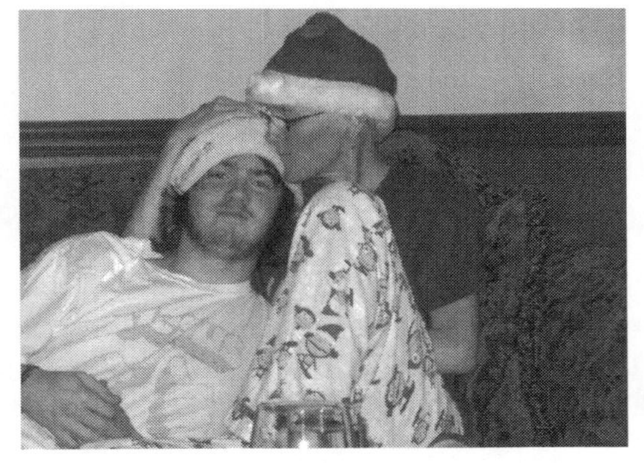

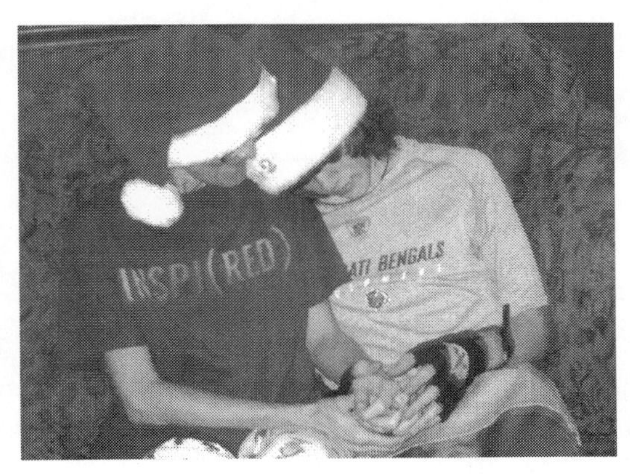
INSPI(RED)
ATI BENGALS

Part of the shakedown of cancer is the in-your-face possibility that this very well might be your last Christmas. It's morbid to think that. I know. But it's kind of hard not thinking it, when you're in the middle of a chemo flight from which you're not sure you'll land safely. So, coupled with an intense desire to make it *the most meaningful* (excluding, of course, the first) *Christmas ever*, just in case, is a dull and seemingly thwarted capacity to really make much ado about *anything*.

So, you make do. About nothing. That's what we did and it was kind of like magic. All of a sudden, I was aware again that I was still here. I was decked with my family all around me, with a cozy fire in the Evanshire, and a real live Christmas tree, all decked out, and yes, there were presents under the tree. It felt more like much ado than nothing. Not merely contentment that this is my lot, but, rather *this is a lot*. Cancer made me appreciate Christmas like I never had before. A backhanded gift, I know, but not all gifts that come in the front door are good. Exhibit A: the horse Odysseus gave to the ancient Greeks. Exhibit B: white elephant gifts. Case closed.

When you have cancer, there is no room for an elephant to hide in the middle of the room. Partially because the lights reflect off of your bald head, making it virtually impossible for even a small cat to hide (let alone the giant white elephant with a fluorescent pink ribbon tattooed on it). And everyone knows a cat can't resist pouncing on a flashing light. Now, I don't know if elephants like to pounce on flashing lights or not, but trust me, they can't hide. The most they can do is pretend to be a screen to show home videos on. But if you look closely, you'll be able to tell. They'll eventually have to blink, or blow their trunk, or swat a fly with their tail (if you happen to have flies on the wall). Also you can throw a mouse into the mix if you don't mind your whole house getting destroyed. Everyone knows elephants are scaredy-cats of mice and they will jump up on a stool if you have one convenient. I recommend having one on hand; otherwise, trust me, that elephant may end up in your lap.

What none of us expected was a bug. A bug can pretty much hide anywhere.

On the second day of Christmas, the bug, which had hitched a ride, and been hiding in Charlie Brown's intestines, came out of hiding. The day after Christmas also happened to be Dave and my twenty-first anniversary. Now, normally twenty-one's a lucky deal, but as you might expect, the tables were turned at the Evanshire. It ended up being more of a crapshoot. Literally. And this is where the dream sequence started getting a little hurly-burly, as the little bug went knocking on the bathroom doors, one by one. People fell like dominos, lined up in rows, where all rows led to the porcelain throne.

First, Charlie Brown . . . then his daddy . . . then my mum. My sister must be part superhero, because somehow she dodged the bug enough to pack their car, sanitize my basement where they'd been staying, and sneak out to buy some Imodium for their impending twelve-hour drive back to Charleston. And they were off. Didn't quite make it all the way in one day, but they were determined to take that damn bug as far away from me as they could before they had to pull over.

Shortly after they left, we checked my mum into a hotel, which had a cleaner B&B (bed and bathroom) for her to catch a little R&R (rest and recuperation) while we tried to contain things around the Evanshire in hopes of keeping the bug at exile's distance. Besides our twenty-first anniversary, it also happened to be Boxing Day. We didn't have any boxing gloves, but we do like to get in the spirit of things, and, well, we did have cleaning gloves, so we improvised. I mean, we already looked like a couple of Mr. Clean clones, so why not go ahead and channel him and get our Evanshire sanitized in one fell swoop?

If that's not a literal clearing of the stage for a romantic twenty-first anniversary celebration, then I don't know what is. If nothing else, then I don't know if there has ever been such a clean stage. Anywhere. We not only set the bar high, we spit-shined and polished it, clean enough to see our own lemontini-fresh mugs in it.

When we finally put down our dukes and gave the Evanshire the Mr. Clean seal of approval, we decided to go buy some lottery tickets. Seriously, we bought twenty-one lottery tickets. Which we quickly turned into thirty lottery tickets. Then it was slowly downhill from there. The thirty turned into seven; the seven turned into four; the four replicated themselves; and then there were none.

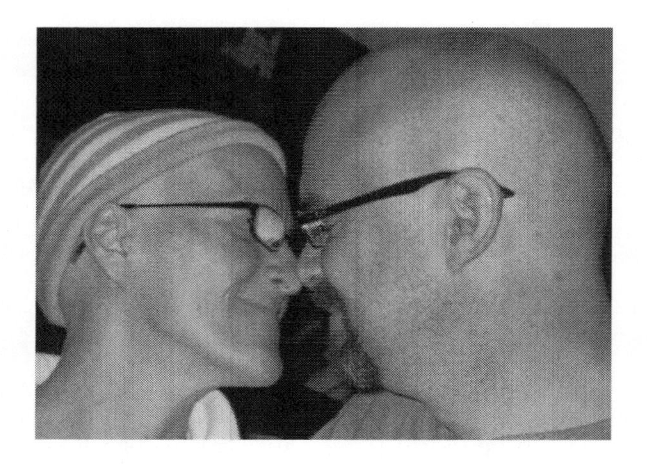

A little Agatha Christie of an ending, but it was fun. We had a cheering section: the workers in the gas station and the guy standing behind us in line. He said he saw someone buy twenty and turn them into five hundred dollars once, so everybody was counting on us winning, so we'd share the love and buy a round of coffee. I'm pretty sure they were also secretly hoping for a Krispy Kreme or two if we won big. One of the girls in the gas station said, "Good luck," as we walked out to our car to scratch off the first batch of lottery tickets while we bought Yukon a drink. I looked at Dave, took off my hat, and said, "I suppose I look like I could use some." We just cracked up, grabbed a couple of dimes (the size of gallstones) from the ashtray, and scratched that itch, for fun and laughter, for the win.

The third and fourth days of Christmas were sort of a blur, because Dave and Mikeyy both caught the bug. As for me, we couldn't tell if the bug or the chemo was to blame. All we knew was theirs was definitely a bug, not chemo.

On the fifth day of Christmas I downed Round 7. This part really was like a dream, because I fell asleep. Unfortunately, a nap was not part of my plan since it was the first time my Redheads came to hang out with me during chemo. I was so excited. We'd packed a picnic of Chipotle burritos, which we munched on during the anti-nausea meds and Tax-ALL drips, all while setting up the "pink" Monopoly game my Uncle Bill had given me. At which point—well, I have to defer to the Redheads on this one, since I guess that Tax-ALL was one too many, because I kind of, sort of, passed out.

Here is their report, in a blog post entitled "Redheads: Taking Over" in which, they hacked my blog:

> Feel the power? Amanda reporting here, and through the brilliance of three combined, adorable Evans heads we've managed to hack Mum's blog. This time the public is going to be blessed by hearing about Mum's life through our mystical and very brown eyes.
>
> Yesterday, being the 29th of December, was a Monday. Everyone knows Mondays are the worst of all days, primarily because they signal the death of a weekend. But in our house, they are even more tragic than that. Mondays. Are. Chemo days. Our lives are systchematically ;) planned around these Mondays. Mum goes through an aggravating cycle of progressively getting healthier until the Chemonday comes and she is shot back down.
>
> This Chemonday Mum had a big send-off into her sick week. For the first time, oddly enough, the whole family came. For once, I was off of school and work and so were my brothers. So the whole family all piled into the Turd Machine aka our smelly brown van, and headed off. It felt like a road trip. We packed iPods, pink Monopoly, and Coke.
>
> OK, Mikeyy here now. It did indeed feel like a road trip, as we embarked on this deadly adventure through Chemotherapy, starring Joules Evans as herself and Dr. Lower as The Oncologist. Guest starring Herceptin and the villain, a mean dose of Taxol. Supporting actors being Dave, Amanda, Matt, and Mikeyy Evans, also helped by the wonderful input of the nurses.
>
> As if the long drive wasn't tough enough, we then had to wait in the waiting room for about thirty minutes. Not the most exciting time, I must assure you. We did, however learn of an excellent sandwich, mixing garlic bread and lasagna, from Paula Dean on the Food Network. Mmm :) Finally, we were called back to go to Dr. Lower's office. Hopes, mostly from us kids, of getting this rocking and rolling were dashed when we were forced to wait in her office for another forty minutes. Finally she came, much to all our relief. She's an interesting one, Dr. Lower. Very cool and nice; she has a teachery-type personality to her. And she rocks because she's saving our mum's life. Anyway, finally, we were off to the upstairs to start this chemo cocktail! We all secretly hoped

> to get a cocktail of our own, though obviously we're not talking the chemo kind.
>
> I guess it's my (Matt's) turn now. I've gotta say, I agree with that whole road trip feeling it had. We had the cooler and games and books and iPods and everything. The car ride just wasn't long enough to quite cut it, but I'm fine with that.
>
> The worst part for me was probably the needles. I like needles just about as much as my mum does. Which is not at all. And some lady kept leaving that biohazard trash box open, which, with all my OCD-ness and stuff wasn't all that great haha =p I had to move to the other side of the room. The waiting was all right. Long, but all right. And other than that we just kind of chilled, played some Monopoly, ate some Chipotle, and watched *Psych* and *That '70s Show*. The doctor and nurses were pretty nice, too. Doctor-office-type places always make me extremely exhausted for some reason or other, so by the time we left (around six-thirty, I think...) I was about ready to go to bed. Even though I didn't. But, yeah.
>
> Mikeyy now, again! Basically, the day was very exhausting for all of us. The chemo place was a little eerie at six. All those dark rooms, and we were the only people left. The day could've been a lot scarier, especially if we were in the big room with everybody else. Luckily, we had a room to ourselves, so it was nice and peaceful. I must confess though: Mum's a snorer on chemo! ;). She's going to kill me now for saying that. Anyway, yeah. It was a rather tiring day, especially for Mum, who first got pierced by needles, then pumped full of anti-nausea meds, Herceptin, and Taxol all day long. Quite tiring. We all escaped alive, however, and will live to fight chemo another day. Mum stands the conqueror, after six heavy hours battling with her shiny sword, Herceptin, and her trusty steed, Taxol. Equipped with other side weapons, she battles on to destroy the cancer. Said cancer's ETD (Estimated Time of Destruction) is December '09. We'll see you there.

The hacking of my blog, and with it, the slanderous claim concerning my supposed "chemo snoring," happened on the sixth day of Christmas, by the way. Talk about geese a-libeling, I mean, a-laying. But, no, I didn't sue my own kids or anything.

I was in the thick of a chemo fog pretty much the sixth through the tenth days of Christmas. That is, up until the part when Dave's gallbladder went into labor in the wee hours of the tenth day. Well, not actual baby-delivering-labor but it was labor intensive, and one way or another, by surgeon or priest, that damn gallbladder needed to be delivered stat. So in another interesting turn of events, I found myself sitting on the waiting room side of things. I'm pretty sure we completely confused the emergency room staff when I, bald-headed and unsteady on my feet, wheeled Dave up to the receptionist's desk.

On the eleventh day of Christmas, a gallbladder surgeon delivered Dave of his galling gallbladder and a gallstone the size of a dime. I doubt Dave will ever tire of telling about the time he was, quite literally, nearly nickeled and dimed to death. I know him pretty well after twenty-one years of marriage. And I also pretty much know his complete joke repertoire by heart as well. It hasn't altered much since he took me out to eat on one of our first dates, and he said, "You're stuffed? And all this time, I thought you were real." Or the time he asked me to pass him the sham-poo, since we didn't have any real-poo, on our honeymoon. And he's been piling it on, as it were, accumulating jokes as if he were "getting his act together," because deep down, he really wants to be a stand-up comedian when he grows up.

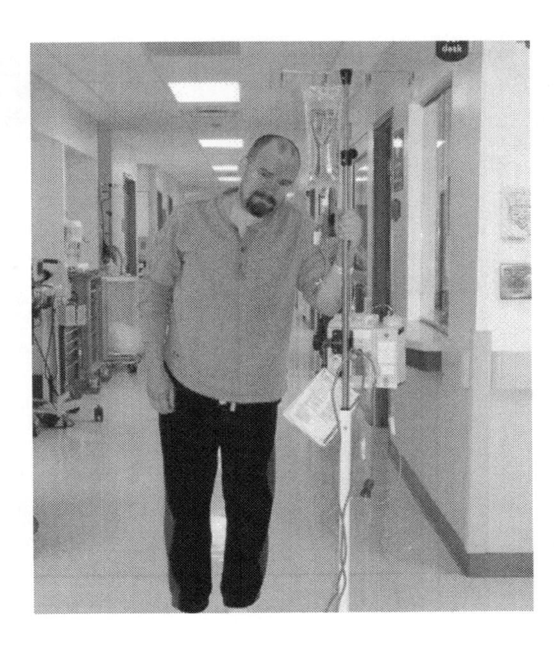

On the twelfth day of Christmas, Dave was home recovering from his surgery, and I was focusing, really hard, on not being so freaking funny around the house. It was out of consideration for him, because he was still sore whenever he laughed. And I especially didn't want to cause him to bust a gut. Literally. That would have made me throw up for sure. Meanwhile, all of a sudden we realized that not only was this the twelfth night, but 2009 had snuck up on us. Whoa. And we were already so over 2008. It felt good to crack open a fresh calendar.

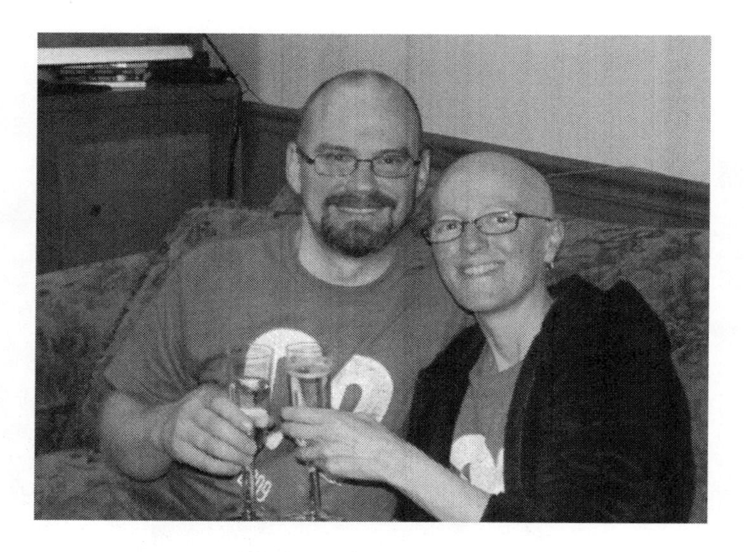

The next day was Epiphany. And how.

Round 8
Only One More Round (of Tax-ALL)

Round 1 of Tax-ALL sucked. I don't really feel like mincing words about it because what's the point? And no, it's not because I'm one of those anti-mincing freaks, just in case you were wondering. The truth is, I actually get into mincing . . . when it's garlic and/or onions. Mincing words when it comes to Tax-ALL, however, is just not my style. But if I could literally mince Tax-ALL—well, I have to admit that I've had dreams about that. I'd totally slice, dice, and karate chop it into a million bajillion times infinity little pieces—if I had my way, after the way it tried to make mincemeat of me. But then again, it also hopefully sucker punched any remaining mutant cancer cells, so you see my dilemma. No mincing at *all* when it comes to Tax-ALL.

Round 2 still sucked, but a little bit less. Sucking is still sucking, and really is only a good thing in reference to vacuum cleaners and anteaters, in which case not sucking means your vacuum's broken or you've got a skinny anteater on your hands.

Round 3 was Round 2's tag-team twin. I won't say the *s* word again here, but I think it's safe to assume that I'm thinking it as I type. Tax-ALL knocked me down like three strikes almost in a row.

Usually that means you're out. Yeah, I know a thing or two about baseball.

I have no idea how I kept getting back up, except that it's really the only thing you can do. There's a saying that when you're knocked down, the only way to look is up, and I've found it to be true. I mean, when you get knocked down, the only things at eye level are feet. I don't know anyone who really likes gazing at dirty feet. Even my daughter, who cures pedis for a living, actually nurses a bit of a foot phobia herself.

Anyway, once I got back up after downing Round 3, I was a little bruised (at least, my feet *felt* like I was walking on bruises, due to the neuropathy I was experiencing from the Tax-ALL pummeling), but I wasn't quite down for the count—though, when I look at pictures now, it looks like you could have TKO'd me if you sneezed in my direction. (Note: never sneeze in a chemo patient's direction, or for that matter, in their vicinity, because they have an impaired immune system; therefore, one person's gesundheit might very well end with another's TKO.) So yeah, I came out swinging, and surprisingly, with my tennis racquet.

Since I couldn't exactly play competitive tennis during the dog days of chemo, I'd go to the club to watch my friends play whenever I'd round the corner to not-a-chemo weeks. It was a way to keep from feeling like I was falling off the planet and out of the loop of my life. Also, I've always been one to believe in the osmosis theory when all else (like your health, fitness, not to mention your entire immune system and muscle tone) fails, so it was actually like tennis practice for me. I definitely learned patience, perspective, strategy, and even technique while sitting on the sidelines, and I think I'm a better player now because of it.

On this particular not-a-chemo week, I dusted off my tennis racquet and took it with me to the club to watch my team practice, just for kicks. I was in a good mood and all, because it was a TGINACW.

I'd had enough of the sad looks my shiny new orange HEAD tennis racquet kept shooting me from the sweet perch I had arranged for it, right next to my brand new orange Adidas Barricades. (One would *think* matching shoes would make a racquet happy.) It was also near my side of the room, where it was practically the first thing I'd see when I woke up and stumbled out of bed. Anyway, after practice I was talking to one of our tennis pros, and next thing I knew she had fed me a whole basket of real live tennis balls! Now, I'm not saying it was pretty, but I hit 'em. My racquet was so happy it could barely stand it. I did feel a bit bad, though, because I didn't bring my new shoes. I don't wear my tennis shoes except on court, and I didn't take them with me because of the ongoing neuropathy in my feet. (They were still feeling soggy and fat, the way Novocain makes your lip feel. They fit in my shoes, but they didn't *feel* like they fit in my shoes, if that makes any sense. But then again, saying my feet felt like a fat lip doesn't make much sense either. I hadn't been wearing shoes as much as possible, let alone *changing* them once I stuffed my soggy feet in them.) The downside to not wearing my shoes was the dejected attitude I had to deal with from my shoes, since my racquet simply could not contain itself once we got home.

It was good therapy all around before going back in the ring for Round 4. Keeping an eye on the bouncing ball is a good focusing technique. Hitting the bouncing ball is classic stress relief therapy.

The only part of Round 4 I was looking forward to was the part where I was done paying the Tax-ALL man. I knew it was going to suck. Fortunately, the night before chemo was Amanda's eighteenth birthday, so celebrate mode faked out dread mode.

Every four years the presidential inauguration falls on Amanda's birthday. January 20, 2009, was one of those years, making it an especially historical one. I was one proud mama, so happy to be there, to sing "Happy Birthday" to my little girl, the newest, not to mention cutest, IMHO, voter on the suffrage scene. Living to see the first African American president and another peaceful transition of power, I was proud to be an American.

We took Amanda out, to one of her *Cheers* places from her high school days, an Indian restaurant we used to live around the corner from called the Taj Mahal. They didn't yell "Norm!" or anything, but whenever she walked in the door, this one particular waiter would always bring her an order of jalabi, which are like coils of fried dough dripping with honey. She has called it "the nectar of the gods," ever since that love at first bite. The waiter seems to get a kick out of her hereby dubbing of the jalabi, because this is the ritual when she walks in the door.

He offers up the jalabi.

She receives it, is pleased.

She hereby dubs it. He smiles and then notices the rest of us, her loyal subjects, and takes our order. After, of course, he brings her a mango lassi to cleanse her palette.

The distraction technique worked like a charm. You would've thought I was Muhammad Ali the way I was dodging the taunting "tomorrow's a chemo Monday" punches. It was as if I was practically dancing around the ring, taunting right back, like I "float like a butterfly, sting like a bee."

There would be no chemo buzz nor sting until the sun rose on another chemo Monday, the next day. So even though I was in celebrate mode, I was conscious on some level that I was still in training for treatment. Which meant, diet and attire for the main event.

My last supper before the last bell rang on Round 4 was chicken tika masala. Since my taste buds were back in the game, I ordered my usual: an eleven, on a scale of one to ten, with ten being the spiciest. I know. *Rocky* did raw eggs. But that is disgusting. Just the thought of guzzling raw eggs makes me want to hurl, and I was trying to keep the hurling at bay. No, for me, a good pre-game appetizer is all about carbs and heat. You know that old saying, "If you can't stand the heat, get out of the kitchen." Well, them's taunting words that seemed to apply here. To which I said, "Bring it!"

Besides a proper meal, it's also important to dress appropriately when you're going in for the fight of your life. As in, a new uniform. Unfortunately, Nike hadn't contacted me quite yet, but luckily, I made it to the Lucky Brand store while I was birthday shopping for Amanda. I bought a T-shirt with a floppy-eared mouse in boxing gloves, with his dukes raised, which seemed appropriate for the occasion of Round 8.

I know, I was supposed to be buying stuff for Amanda, but how could I not buy that T-shirt? It practically had my name written all over it. I felt a little like a mouse sometimes, fighting cancer and dealing with chemo. And it wasn't the first time the analogy had been drawn. When I was growing up, and playing a mean shortstop on my softball team, my teammates used to call me Mighty Mouse whenever I was at bat. How perfect was this T-shirt?

Except for one minor detail. Turns out, it was actually a rabbit, not a mouse, on the shirt.

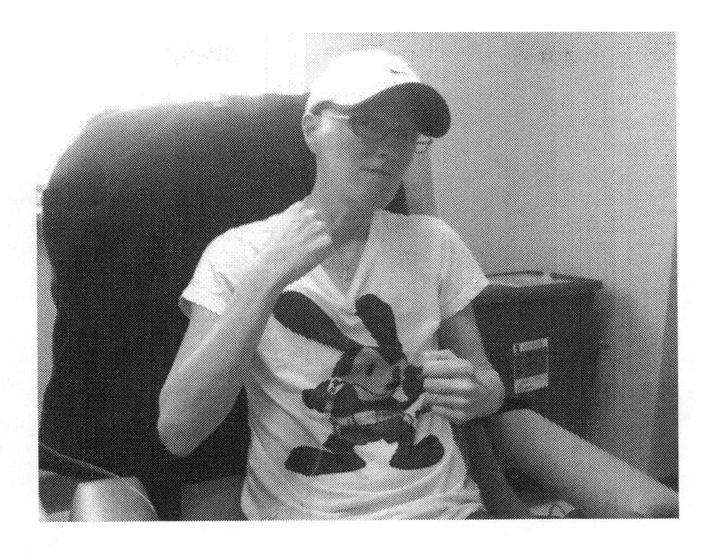

Oops. Blame that one on the chemo for sure. What gave it away was the fine print right above the *rabbit's* left foot that says, "Oswald: Lucky Rabbit." So that wasn't even my name written all over it, either. Whatever. Anyway, at first this was all a bit of a downer, because a lucky rabbit's foot is most commonly detached from said rabbit—and hanging on a key chain—while the poor rabbit is, well, I don't even want to go there. But at the very least, I wouldn't call him lucky. And that wouldn't exactly be the encouraging message I was trying to convey when I suited up in that T-shirt for my last round of Tax-ALL. But then, I thought about it really hard, and decided that it was indeed a lucky rabbit since he was still standing on *both* lucky feet in the picture.

Which is exactly what I was trying to do.

Round 9
Sweet Dreams

After I slammed down my last taxing Tax-ALL chemo cocktail, I pretty much slept off the weekend, as per my usual, to try to stay ahead of the pain curve.

I was leaning forward, *Titanic*-style, hoping to turn the corner, sticking out my neck like a triple-crown champ, toward feeling better. By Monday morning of TGINACW, I thought I had turned the corner. But I must have been dreaming, because late Monday night I turned one corner and ran smack dab into another corner. This was a most unfortunate turn of events. I felt like a big, fat bruise, sore to the touch. In fact I was even a little sore if you looked at me wrong. I was cranky as all get out. (Just ask my kids.) I had one helluva headache; two numb, swollen, freezing cold feet; and ten numb, fumbling fingers that couldn't really feel the keys on my computer—yet I had an uncanny ability to feel sorry for myself. I was quite disappointed to find myself in what I could only assume was some kind of evil polygon, with all sorts of convoluted corners, instead of the simple, if obtuse, angle I *thought* I was dealing with. Have I mentioned that I suck at math? (Cue the needle scratching across the record special effect and, well, so much for the *Titanic* theme song in the background.) Yes, I am quite aware that was a bit melodramatic. Sorry. I got carried away. It's that song. But in case you were worrying about me, since you are probably just the kind of gentle reader to do something sweet like that, I wasn't really wallowing in my misery, if that's the way it sounds. I was dog paddling my way through it, to get to the other side.

The other side is always worth it. And it's especially nice if there's somebody who's already been there, done that, bought the T-shirt cheering you on as you paddle away.

Like the kind woman who gently tapped me on the shoulder in the mannequin hand aisle at Sally Beauty Supply where Amanda and I were on a scavenger hunt. We were checking off a list (and filling a cart in the process), shopping for supplies she needed to take the Ohio state boards to get her nail tech license. I'm sure we had passed the mannequin hands so many times in the course of our beauty shop bingo that to the casual observer it might have appeared as if all those fake fingers kept pointing us away from themselves. The truth is we both like crossing off lists and we were trying to remember where in the world the mannequin hands were . . . when I felt the tap, tap, tapping on my shoulder. Talk about *bingo*! I practically peed my pants.

"So, you're a survivor."

Yeah, that shocked me a bit, too. But the part that shocked me the most was my response, which surprisingly was not me doing a Scooby-Doo, screaming, "Zoinks!" while jumping into Amanda's arms, which were busy grabbing a mannequin hand anyway.

"Yeah, I guess I am." I turned around and we two survivors met "eye of the tiger" to "eye of the tiger."

She met me with a wink and a smile and without missing a beat said, "I could tell because I used to have the same hairstyle."

Then she told me her story about how she had been diagnosed with a breast cancer very similar to mine a few years ago, and how she had received very similar treatments: Herceptin, being a most happy and hopeful similarity. The difference was that her diagnosis was stage 4, and the prognosis she'd been given was . . . gulp . . . not good. But, there she was, with hair down to her shoulders and a helping hand—tapping on my shoulder, calling *me* a survivor. Like I was one of the gang. Wow.

Then she just raved about my eyebrows. They were, at that point, mostly, still there. And still mocking me about the time I let Amanda coax me into "voluntarily" having them ripped from my forehead only to find out that they would have un-furrowed on their own once

I was up to my eyes in chemo cocktails. Poor eyebrows. There they were, perfectly happy, minding their own business, dotting eyes and connecting the dots. Not bothering anyone, really.

Now eyebrows remind me of that generous soul who took the time to tap on my shoulder in the middle of the mannequin hand aisle. It was as if she pointed out the lovely view from the other side of cancer and tossed me a rope from the other side of chemo. She taught me that eyebrows are worth raving about.

I also had a couple of eyelashes left. But we didn't go there. I think we both knew it might have gotten a little out of control in the middle of the mannequin hand aisle and we might have gotten thrown out of the store or something. And then who would do my nails?

The other side of Round 9 was also going to be something to rave about. Not that chemo was all of a sudden fun or anything. But I was done with the mis- part of the treatment. And I didn't miss that misplaced syllable one bit. Now, it was just plain old treatment. Or I guess, if we're being technical, fancy new treatment. Things seemed to be looking up with Herceptin flying solo in the cocktail pit.

For one thing, I wouldn't need anti-nausea meds in my chemo cocktail any longer, since Herceptin isn't normally associated with the nasty side effects of traditional chemotherapy. This meant less drip time in the chemo cocktail lounge.

I wouldn't have to take anti-nausea meds every six hours for three days after, either. Part of me wondered if Dave was going to miss being my alarm clock/pharmacist. What in the world was he going to do with all that spare time? I hoped he wouldn't get any ideas about picking up extra shifts as my personal trainer, either out of boredom or having gotten used to telling me what to do with me being so on drugs, I mean, so easygoing, about it.

I wouldn't have to come back every Tuesday after chemo Monday to get the Neulasta shot, either. No more traditional chemo meant we were no longer in seek-and-destroy mode. Herceptin was immune therapy, so not only had the teardown been completed, it was time to build up.

That. Sounded. Good. So good.

One more thing: no more MiraLAX. One of the crappiest things about chemo, not to mention pain meds, is that they are incredibly horribly constipating. Besides the thrush trauma of my first round of chemo, there was also the trauma of not going to the bathroom for a week. I was so literally full of shit it almost scared the shit out of me, except I couldn't. I've never been one who goes around talking about bathroom functions and such, so it's not exactly my favorite thing that some of my best advice about chemo has to do with constipation. But seriously, I don't know how a cancer/chemo memoir can leave out this other *C* word. It may be foul to speak about such things, but constipation is just as much of a bitch as the other two *C*'s.

What finally worked for me was lacing my coffee with MiraLAX on cheMonday morning. It's not supposed to have a taste, but it does—though, it's not the worst thing in the world. Constipation, on the other hand, might be the worst thing in the world. So all you can do is go with it, or, you might not ever go, if you know what I mean. I'd also add MiraLAX to a cup of chamomile tea before bed cheMonday night.

I'd repeat this every day and night of chemo week, and usually by day 4 or so, I was "not full of shit" anymore. At which point I would put the brakes on the MiraLAX, as the opposite effect would kick in at that point if I wasn't careful. It really is quite a precise balancing act one must perform in the midst of the fog of chemo.

My body didn't quite trust me going in to Round 9. Against my will and in the face of reason, my body tensed up every time the phone rang on Thursdays before cheMondays, just anticipating the chemo reminder call. Even though I knew that this round would be different, better, it's not like my body would even listen. Who could blame it? It's hard to win some*body*'s trust back. These things take time. At least Round 9 was a step in the right direction.

Beyond the new and improved protocol, there were two other important baby steps: First, I just said no—no chemo nap, no chemo hangover, and no bucket nearby. I was awake, alert still, at nine p.m., and aware enough to wonder why there wasn't a new *House* episode on, so maybe my going clean would rub off on Dr. House and maybe he'd kick the Vicodin. Now that I knew Vicodin intimately, I couldn't help but have nightmares worrying about how constipated the poor guy had to be.

The second step (drumroll, please) was that I had a real live hair day!

I have to say that it was probably good my mum lives out of town, because she used to love taping bows to my head. (She says she did this so people would know I was a little girl since I had nothing but peach fuzz until I was two years old.) I wouldn't have put it past her to try those old shenanigans again. But, I'm not much more of a bow kind of girl now than I was back then. Of course this all meant I'd have to think about shaving my legs again. The bright side to that was that my razor would be a useful little razor and therefore happy once again.

Besides bringing my razor out of retirement, it was time to start rebuilding this bionic woman. Or maybe putting Humpty Dumpty together again is more appropriate. Regardless, I'd begun working out toward regaining my fitness. There were quite a few muscles that had been hibernating during the winter of my discontent. I'm pretty sure they made that bionic sound and everything when I tried to wake them up. Yeah, it was slow-mo, but it was bionic. "We'll make her stronger. Faster. Able to leap tall buildings in a single bound." Well, something along those lines.

That first week I swam laps twice, hit tennis balls once, took a two-mile walk, and worked out with some hand weights. Not bad for a first week back. I was a tiny bit surprised that Nike hadn't called to sponsor my comeback yet. I was excited to wear the swoosh in an official capacity, but then it totally made sense to me that they might rather have somebody who already "just did it" be encouraging everyone to "just do it" instead of some rookie "wanna do it." So I didn't mind "just doing it" anyway, even without my own line of clothing, or Nike officially on my team.

What I didn't expect, though, was losing one of the most significant cheerleaders in my life, at this crucial time in my life: my grandma, or Gramcracker as I called her. I don't remember exactly when I started calling her Gramcracker. Somewhere along the road, I got taller, *relatively* speaking, as in, taller than *her*; and I guess I just felt like my cute little grandma needed a special pet name. "Gramcracker" just rolled off my tongue like it was destiny. I wish there was s'more to it, but there's not.

Her given name was Gloria, which means glory. It doesn't surprise me that she didn't go by it, though. I don't know all her reasons, but I like to imagine that she gave her given name to God, just like she lived, for his own glory. She went by Eileen, which means *light*, and makes total sense if you knew her. When she was a little girl, and shortly after she started speaking, she called herself, I-E.

At twenty-one months, she was saying her prayers. Begging her mum to read the Bible to her about Jesus. Begging her mum to sing hymns to her. (I use the word *begging* in the loosest sense of the word, if you think her mum actually had any choice, and only because *begging* is the euphemism her mum wrote in her baby book. If you knew my Gramcracker, you read that word more like an antonym.) At two-years-old, two of her favorite songs were "Jesus Bids Us Shine" and "Jesus Wants Me for a Sunbeam." So. Fitting. For a little girl called light.

Once when she was sick, she *begged* her mom and grandma to sing those hymns to her, over and over, again and again, until they were almost sick but literally tired of them. And, probably hoarse—if I know my Gramcracker.

Come to think of it, maybe the name was more of a divine tip than a mere slip of the tongue. Grandma plus firecracker equals Gramcracker. By the time she was four years old, she put childish things and prayers aside, preferring to say The Lord's Prayer before bedtime rather than the "little" one her little brother said. From a very young age, I-E seemed to embody her name. Almost as if the children's song "This Little Light of Mine" was written just for her.

She graced my life with her godly presence and prayers from the moment I was born until the Thursday night she went home to be with God and my grandpa. That is 15,845 days that she was my example and 15,845 days that she prayed for me. One of the most significant and beautiful things anybody has ever done or will ever do for me. It humbles me and lifts me up all at the same time. And makes me feel very, very blessed. And, yes, Josh Groban is singing "You Raise Me Up" in the background of my mind right now when I think about it.

I count it a blessing that I was able to visit her in the hospital before she went to be with God. I hadn't been able to see her since before I was diagnosed with breast cancer in August; neither of us was in a condition to travel. She had a fall near the end of January and ended up in the hospital. The nasty fall ended up being a nastier domino: a slight fracture in her pelvis, terrible bruising on her arms, edema in her legs and feet, congestive heart failure, low blood pressure, digestive issues, a series of mini-strokes, and delirium. All this was complicated by a heart murmur and the fact that she was quite hard of hearing. I had just downed my last "bad" chemo cocktail and thankfully, when I turned the corner from it, Amanda and I were able to visit her in the hospital.

When I walked in the room, she started crying and said she had been worried that she might not ever get to see me again. Then she proceeded to worry about me getting sick by coming to the hospital. She said she didn't want her sufferings to add to my own. Which was very much like her, but the last thing on my mind. We had a lovely visit. She was in good spirits. We chatted back and forth with the help of a little whiteboard that I wrote on. I was never good at yelling things to my Gramcracker like my mum and aunties were. I never could even bring myself to try it. The whiteboard was more up my alley, and I think I got to say everything I wanted to. I hope I brought her some comfort and cheer. Before we left, with Dave and the boys on speakerphone, Amanda and I laid hands on her, and we all prayed over her. We laid the phone next to her good ear; I'm pretty sure she somehow heard all the prayers, because she seemed to be leaning into them and to be soothed by them. I keep playing that day over and over again in my head, and it was perfect. My sister and cousins all had similar moments with her on the phone where, looking back, we all knew she was saying her goodbyes. I sensed it, from the first words she said to me when I walked in the door, to the last ones before I left, when she was telling me that I could have anything of hers that I wanted.

She suffered so much those last couple of weeks in the hospital that it broke our hearts. I think she knew she was dying and I think she was ready. Characteristically, she did it like a faithful servant of God, and on her own terms that she had with him.

She said her goodbyes, making sure she left everyone feeling like they were her favorite. She tried to give all her stuff away. One day she told my Auntie Cheryl to give her clothes and canned food to the mission my husband's brother runs. Cheryl asked her what in the world she thought she was going to wear when she got out of the hospital. Without missing a beat, my Gramcracker said they could just put a towel around her! This was my Gramcracker, and not terribly unlike my grandpa, who, when he went before her a few years earlier, had requested that we bury him in his bathrobe. An interesting reunion, to say the least. Yes, I came by all this honestly.

Having said her goodbyes, she rolled up her sleeves, fixed her eyes on Jesus, and suffered everything that came her way until he wrapped things up and then took her in his arms.

My Gramcracker is not suffering any more.

Those are some of the words I spoke at her funeral. To me, her life was what sweet dreams are made of. She traveled the world and found what she was looking for. And may she rest in peace.

Rounds 10 through 12
Wind in My Hair

Sometimes I know I act like I think the world revolves around me. This revelation probably doesn't surprise you, since you're sitting here reading my memoir. Or at least I hope you're sitting here reading it, and not making paper airplanes[40] out of the pages, or using them to line your birdcage.[41] The latter one especially would hurt my feelings, because it reminds me of when my sister and I used to have birds, and Pepler (my bird) kept eating all the bird food, and poor Lemonade (her bird) ended up next to Woodstock on the Snoopy comic strip lining the cage.

Anyway, reality checks always make me have one of those V8 moments where I realize things are askew and I slap myself on the forehead. I totally get it that everything's not all about me. (Even this memoir really isn't all about me, myself, and I.) And we're all, actually, quite good with that.

It's not that I feel like being the center of the universe anyway, because that's way more pressure than I'm personally comfortable with. Even being the center of attention makes me feel super awkward. Whenever people look at me too long I sort of feel like I might as well be the incarnation of the original faux pas. My first thought is always, "Now what did I go and do?" Then I wonder what my face is doing. Am I smiling? At which point I completely forget how to smile. Then of course I get all worried there's a booger in my nose, or something in my teeth. Which always reminds me of Roseanne Roseannadanna. Which always cracks me up. And when you think about it, standing in a roomful of people while laughing to yourself is not the most socially acceptable behavior in the world either. At which point we've come full circle. Well, like Roseanne Roseannadanna used to always say, "It's always something" now, isn't it?

All that to say, I get distracted kind of easily, because my frame of reference is obviously limited to my own skin and I'm only five-foot-three when I stand as tall as I can. So I hope you can understand why I'm sometimes accidentally preoccupied with myself. It's not my favorite flaw, and if you don't mind, I'd like to change the subject.

This seems like a perfect time to segue into a couple of things that happened at the hospital the last time I saw my Gramcracker that I didn't mention in the eulogy. And as far as segues go, I think you'll agree that this is as smooth a move of a transition as they come.

Gramcracker had one of the most infectious laughs in the whole world. I loved the way her chin and triceps jiggled when she giggled. Apparently she did too, because she was always making jokes and cracking herself up. The last time I saw her, as I explained in the eulogy, she was so happy to see me that she cried, because we hadn't gotten to see each other since I was diagnosed with cancer. She hadn't known if she'd ever see me again before she entered her sweet dreams. But that was only half of the story.

My sweet little old Gramcracker also told me that she was so happy to see me she shit. Literally. Now, this is a bigger deal than you might initially think. See, she had a slightly irrational fear of constipation. When she was a little girl, a cousin of hers died from complications due to constipation. I guess it "impacted" her reason when she became a sweet little old Gramcracker. So much so that Pepto-Bismol was practically one of her four basic food groups. I don't think she minds me writing about it. She's probably still laughing hysterically over that last joke she told me anyway. So, my poor Gramcracker's worst-case scenario, unfortunately happened. Until I arrived on the scene, at which point she was so happy to see me, she wasn't constipated anymore. Part of me isn't sure what to make of that. But, most of me just really loved to see her laugh.

The other thing about the last time I saw my Gramcracker was that she kissed my bald head, and in retrospect I'm pretty sure that's when my hair started growing again.

When I walked into my Brit Lit class the following Monday morning, who would've expected to find a real life Mrs. Potato Head sitting on my desk sprouting grass out of her head? Knowing my class, I should've seen it coming. But there she was, my very own private Idaho aka pet spud, sporting a practical mirror image of me and my new 'do. I named her Ida.

The thing about Ida was that she was a bit of a show-off with her unruly locks. They needed to be mowed, if you want to know the truth. But, I don't mean to come off like sour grapes. I only mentioned it to sketch the character accurately for you, dear reader. What did get on my nerves though, was the incessant batting of her eyelashes. That was just cruel. And, after being so prompted, I had Amanda do an eyelash count: I was down to three! Put yourself in my place and try not to take your pet spud constantly batting her eyelashes at you personally.

The fact that Ida's hair was green and it was almost St. Patrick's Day was just rubbing it in. My hair was translucent, at best, going into Round 10. It was still a lot like peach fuzz.

The nice thing about having peach fuzz for hair was that it was so downy soft my kids felt like they had to pet my head every time they came near me.

I didn't mind.

At first it came in blonde blond, like a towhead. Almost white. You had to catch it in just the right light, or you might miss it.

After the fourth Herceptin I had another MUGA scan to see how my heart was handling the Herceptin. I would have one every three months while on Herceptin. Since the drug is so powerful, it can affect the way the heart pumps. I got the thumbs up. Also, I was radioactive again, with a chance of superpowers, for three more days, to boot.

Besides all that good news, I went into Round 10 with the sudden realization that it had been six months since my mastectomy. That felt like such an amazing milestone. It wasn't a Kodak moment kind of a milestone or anything but more of a pedal-to-the-metal moment. What a rush to see the widening gap (the cleavage of time, if you will) between me and my mastectomy in the rearview mirror. No way was I going to stop or turn around. I just wanted to watch it get smaller and smaller, waving goodbye to the tilted windmills, Rocinante and me.

The only kink going into Round 10 was the gnawing one in my tennis game. Besides the challenge of navigating the court with soggy feet, wet noodle-y legs that had lost both tone and sock tan, there was also the pain in my pec from Port Rafa. It made me wonder if I'd ever be able to serve again. (Or pat my poor pitiful self on the back whenever I felt a little sorry for myself.) There was also a pre-existent tennis rotator cuff issue that I'd hoped six months of inactivity would've helped. Nope. Instead, it seemed to have awakened with the vengeance of a pinched nerve that made my whole right arm feel like it was stuck in a light socket. I'd played with it in my b.c. days, with the aid of copious amounts of Advil to help me just suck it up and play. Not playing tennis didn't really occur to me. I thought starting over from scratch was a big enough challenge. But I'd even fallen behind that curve.

The main difference between Rounds 10 and 11 was one we actually measured with a ruler. An eighth of an inch, to be exact. It was March 10, and I had been having what I can only describe as a good hair day. You can imagine how shocking it must have felt, after having no hair at all since October, nor especially, having that darn double cowlick to contend with all my days before chemo.

I was brushing my teeth that morning when I accidentally looked up, and my first thought was, "Hey, what's Annie Lennox doing here?" All of a sudden she started singing "Sweet Dreams" into the toothbrush she was holding. You might think that since I was standing there with the very same toothbrush in my hand, it would have been more than enough to clue me in. But I had no idea I could dance like that. Also, in my defense, it was before I'd had my coffee.

On my way downstairs to grab some coffee, I happened to look up as I walked past the mirror in the downstairs bathroom. When I saw what looked like my pastor's crazy, white hair shining in the mirror, like a halo or something, I said "Whoa! Dave Workman must've stopped by for coffee. But I wonder why he doesn't shut the bathroom door when he stands in front of the mirror making faces like that?"

As soon as I finished my second cup of coffee, I was thinking clearer, and had a sneaky suspicion.

"Miiii-KEYY!" I interrupted him in the middle of geometry, drawing him from one proof to another. "Can you please bring me that wooden ruler in my desk?"

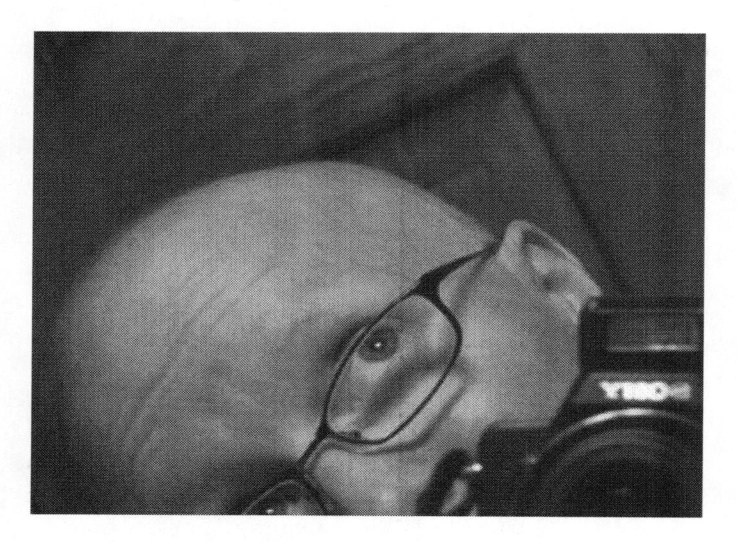

It wasn't Annie Lennox after all; I *can* dance! Also, my hair was officially an eighth of an inch long. One stray strand was even a quarter of an inch! Mikeyy was so proud of me that I thought for sure he was going to grab the pencil from behind my ear and start a growth chart on the kitchen wall, right next to his. Yeah, he's cute like that.

Anyway, at that moment I decided I'd better keep my mad dance moves to myself, to keep it straight who's who between Annie and me. So, if you ever see me dancing and you think, "WTF?" Well, that's why.

I also began physical therapy in between Rounds 10 and 11. I was amped-up nervous about it; after all therapy and torture both start with the letter *t*. Turns out, though, physical therapy's not exactly torture. It wasn't exactly what I'd call fun, either, though. It definitely wasn't as fun as, say, playing tennis. But it wasn't as horrible as having my drains removed either. If I had to go on the record with Greta about it, I'd say it ranked right up there with having my eyebrows waxed.

The main difference between Rounds 11 and 12 can be summed up in a story that begins like a joke: So a chemo patient and her college-age daughter walk into a bar. It's spring break, and they run into a bohemian college prof lady, and it's definitely five o'clock or something, because she says to me, "I love your haircut!"

It was Amanda's spring break and we'd gone south of the border for a girls' weekend away. By south of the border, I'm not talking Mexico, but a little closer to home, in Kentucky, where the grass is blue. We both needed a break, but the furthest road trip I could manage was to a spa hotel a couple of hours away. We had lemon-sugar body scrubs and pedicures, and watched Audrey Hepburn movies all weekend. Probably the highlight of the weekend, though, was washing my hair. I'd only dreamed of using that old excuse, "Sure, I'd like to [insert activity] but I'm busy washing my hair."

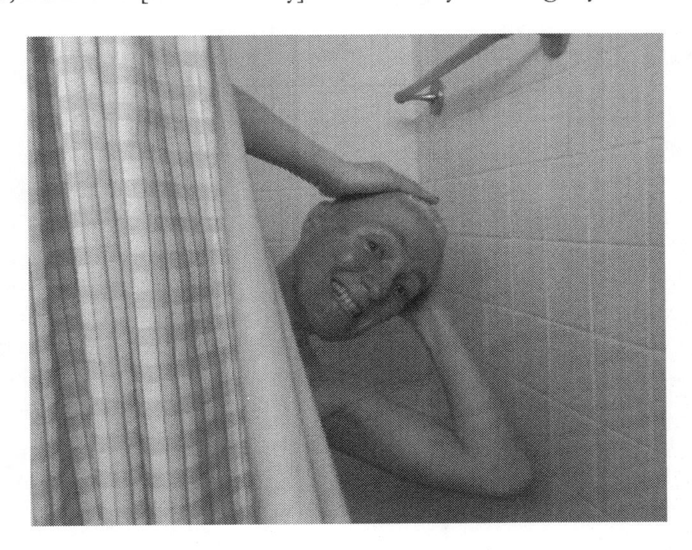

You'd probably get excited too, if your shampoo bottle had been sitting there, all melancholy, since October, making you feel like you don't care or something. I kept trying to cheer it up during its lonely months on the shelf, telling it over and over again that it shouldn't take these things personally. I even told it that I totally thought of it as "half-full." But it was acting like such a melancholy bottle of shampoo, almost to the point of being pessimistic. It wasn't like I didn't already have my hands full, dealing with my hairbrush and my razor, both of which were also clamoring for my attention.

Obviously caught up in the excitement of it all, Amanda decided to have an extreme spa experience, and had her armpits waxed. All I can say was thank God I wasn't in a position to be bullied into what I considered just a step above physical therapy on the pain scale. Personally, I didn't think it was worth the twenty-five dollars it cost, nor the three weeks of no shaving she got in the deal. But then again, I hadn't shaved since October, so I didn't have much room to talk. And I didn't bring it up because I didn't feel like bragging.

When we got back to our room though, I did do an armpit check, and was shocked, to say the least, to find that spring had indeed sprung. I shaved right then and there. Of course, I hadn't packed my own razor, because who would've thunk? So I had to borrow Amanda's. She wouldn't need it for at least three weeks anyway. My only regret was that my own razor had been waiting so patiently up to that point. I wasn't sure how it would take the news. And I didn't trust our shampoo bottle not to make a big scene about it.

On the treatment front, no news was pretty much good news in regard to Rounds 10 through 12. It was also pretty boring as far as chemo cocktails go, and since I don't feel like being boring, I'll finish with another story.

Once upon a time, I woke up with bed-head. And it was a very good hair day. The end. (Note: When I just said "the end" right there, it was just a figure of speech, and not *the* end of the book. It was just the end of that particular story within this bigger story, and not the end, therefore, of this book. So please continue to turn pages and read until *the end,* which will come when you get to the inside of the back cover. In other words, please don't rush out the door and head to Half-Price Books. Not yet. Otherwise, you'll just leave me hanging, before I get to the happily-ever-after part.)

---

[40] http://www.10paperairplanes.com/

[41] A little bonus for the bottom of your birdcage!

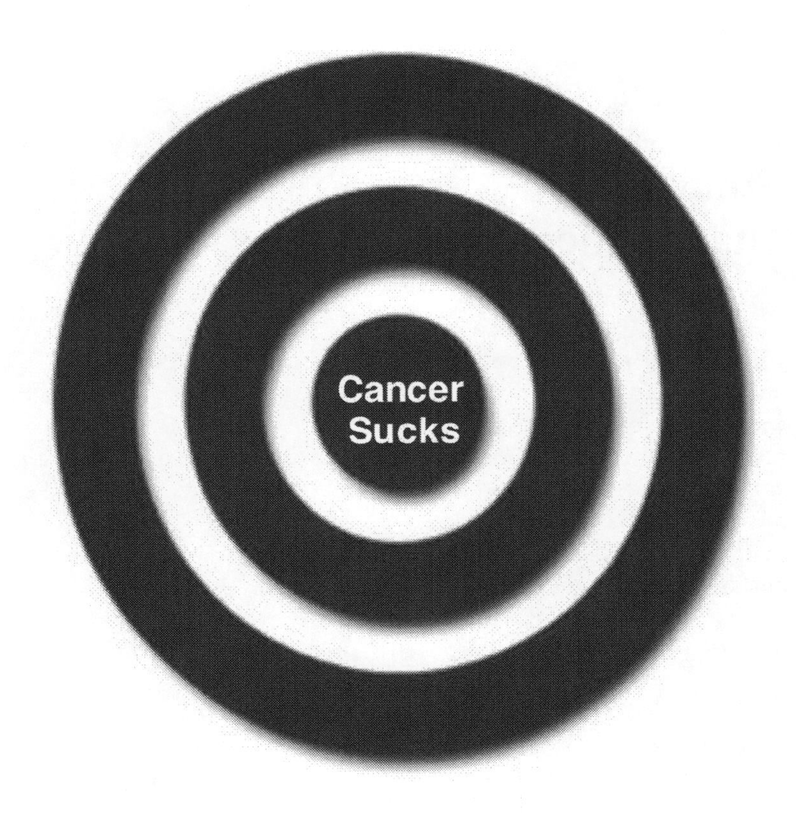

Round 13
That's Amore

Once I'd downed twelve of twenty-four chemo cocktails, it felt like the score was 40-love. I tried not to get all cocky and lose my edge, but I knew I was going to win this match. I knew I still had twelve to down, but I could almost taste the champagne toast after winning the last point and jumping over the net, so why not go ahead and uncork it now?

That's a philosophy I learned from one of my favorite philosophy books: *French Women Don't Get Fat: The Secret of Eating for Pleasure* by Mireille Guiliano. I know it may not be your typical philosophy book, but you're probably not surprised that it's mine. One of my take-aways from the book was that I changed my ways in regard to reserving champagne for special occasions, like anniversaries, New Year's Eve, and yacht christenings. (By that crazy logic, if I never own a yacht, then will there be one less bottle of champagne in my life? I think not.) French women and those who know the secret of eating for pleasure serve champagne as an aperitif. It opens the palate. Part of the thrill of champagne is the delicious irony that the culmination is in the anticipation. In other words, the popping of the cork is like the advent of the dinner.

Speaking of anniversaries, Dave and I had been talking about re-booking the plane tickets we'd had on hold ever since my mastectomy so rudely pulled the old tablecloth out from under our Caribbean holiday. Dr. Lower wasn't crazy about me being barefoot (and practically bare-headed) in the sun, so we booked a Roman holiday where I could eat, pray, love instead. In Rome, my food pyramid would consist of pasta, wine, pizza, gelato, and espresso, and I'd be eating for pleasure like nobody's business.

Dave has always told me that he thinks I have tomato sauce running in my veins and since he was still in carb-loading-me mode, all roads seemed to lead to Rome. I'd always wanted to have my *own* little Roman holiday. But that's not all that was included in this spectacular vacation package: the Tennis World Tour Masters tournament series was headed to Rome the very same week. I asked Dr. Lower if she'd OK me to go the week before Round 13, to mark the twelve I'd downed, and as sort of a bracer for the twelve I still had to go. "Of course!" she said. "OK! Go!" Dr. Lower is probably the most positive, encouraging oncologist in the history of the world. Her philosophy was more like, "Of course you should go on a Roman holiday! Why *wouldn't* you go? Duh."

OK, so maybe she didn't exactly say duh. It's not like she gave me a literal thumbs up either, but lucky for me I have a good imagination. Basically, I took it as a similar prescription to the one Audrey Hepburn's doctor gave her in *Roman Holiday*: "The best thing I know is to do exactly what you wish for a while." Exactly.

I could see that my champagne glass runneth over.

Never mind that I was in the midst of another medical time-out from my own tennis game—doctor's orders—to rest up my lame arm. That was a minor detail. I was going to Rome! Forget that I'd been seeing a physical therapist three times a week, which wasn't as fun as champagne, even though it was *supposed* to be an aperitif to my tennis. How about no therapy for ten delightfully decadent days—in Rome! And that shoulder X-ray—and those MRI findings showing tendinosis in my rotator cuff, arthritis in my clavicle and shoulder, and a fraying of the bursa sac under my biceps tendon. Those were just speed bumps on my way back onto the courts, not to mention, Rome! The surprising part of the report was what I *didn't* have: tennis elbow. That cracked me up a little. But you probably wouldn't believe me if I did have it anyway because that would have been *way* too obvious.

I also *didn't* have more cancer, which was the best kind of news.

My physical therapist followed up that good report with even more good news. It was time to bring my tennis racquet to physical therapy! She said she wanted to see me swing, I mean, to monitor my shoulder during my swing. Then she tossed me a NERF ball, which I figured was due to the fact that she was nervous stepping across the net, so to speak, from me. I thought that was cute, and tried to not let it go to my head. It also helped me remember to take it easy on her, because I didn't feel like intimidating my physical therapist when she was making such progress. (This was the only time physical therapy verged on fun. I think if she'd brought the NERF ball on the first visit, it would have sold the whole physical therapy experience a little better.) Anyway, she ended up giving me the green light to hit nice easy forehands and backhands, no overheads and non-competitively, of course, if I could manage it.

If I could manage it. I couldn't wait to get on the court and "manage it."

It probably won't surprise you that I had a wee tiny bit of a hard time with that non-compete clause. That Friday turned out to be too nice a day not to play tennis outside. The courts behind the Evanshire looked like they needed a bit of cheering up after the winter of their disuse. So I called a few of my tennis girlfriends, and Mikeyy and I headed down my tennis path and to the courts, to just hit around, nothing serious. For about five minutes.

I accidentally ended up playing three sets and getting sunburned in Cincinnati—in April. You probably want to know the scores. Yeah, I got beat. All three sets. The scores were 3-6, 3-6, 3-6. That is, if you like hearing about chemo patients getting beat and stuff. Anyway, despite getting beat, the sunburn, and the fact that I could barely move the next day, the tennis was as priceless as if it were a MasterCard commercial. Which got me to wondering if MasterCard would mind sharing me with Nike. I for one felt there was more than enough me to go around.

What might surprise you, though, was what happened on my Roman holiday. First of all, let me remind you this is a memoir—*not* a novel. The reason I mention it is because I'm worried you're going to throw my book across the room in disbelief when you get to the twist in the plot that's coming soon: my remake of the Audrey Hepburn classic.

I once threw *The Grapes of Wrath* across the room when I got to the last scene. Did not see that coming. Not in a million years. I don't know if I threw it more because it was so disturbing (which was clearly Steinbeck's intent, to afflict the comfortable so we'd snap out of our complacency and be more decent human beings, the kind that comfort the afflicted) or because it was too incredulous. I just couldn't wrap my head around the story going there, no matter how hard I tried, nor how much I admired his mastery for provoking such a profound reaction to his novel. In the end I was just glad I didn't hit anyone with the book and further prove his point. Even if my bad example was more believable than Rose of Sharon's good one. But I digress.

My point is that my final scene in *my* Roman holiday is not a work of fiction. Seriously, I have a pretty cool imagination, but I don't think I could twist a plot like that and get away with it.

OK, so now I'm getting all nervous that I've gone and built it up way too much and that you're going to feel let down when you're finally ready to read what happened.

So, the first thing we did after crossing the pond was to park ourselves at a sidewalk café. We ordered a couple of espressos to counteract the jet lag. Once the caffeine kicked in we headed straight over to the Trevi Fountain and tossed some coins in to make a wish to return to Rome.

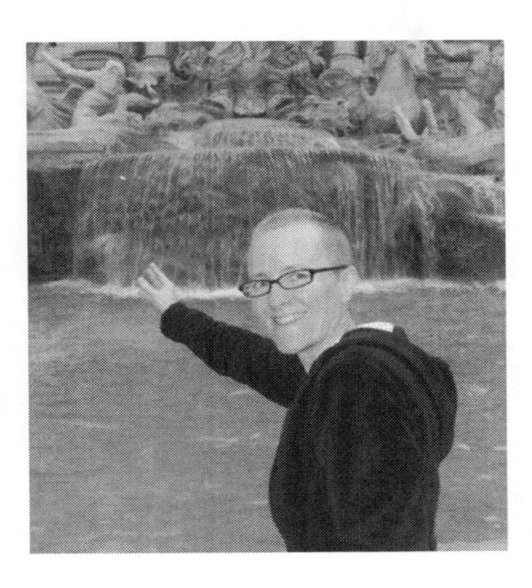

I'd never been there before, but I already knew I was destined to fall in love with the eternal city forever, and already I couldn't wait to come back to Rome, sweet Rome.

I didn't think about it at the time, but just like Audrey, I'd sort of gotten a new hairdo before my Roman holiday. Needless to say, that was unintentional on my part.

To prove I wasn't being a complete copycat, in the absolute sense, I shook things up by tossing in a little Elizabeth Gilbert and eating a whole pizza. Quite a few times, just to get the scene right, even though we weren't in Napoli. I just imagined I was. OK, I threw in quite a lot of that eating part, if you want to know the truth. Who doesn't want to experience spaghetti like that?

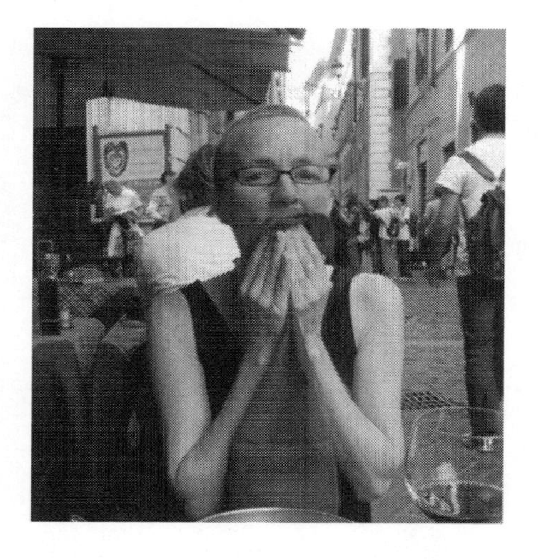

And it was amore at first bite. Love in any language, really. I found my eating center. And I found quite a few cute little apartments with balconies orbiting Piazza Navona that I sure wouldn't mind subletting, so I could keep this balance.

The thing that knocked me off my feet about Rome was that you'd be walking down la via, looking in shop windows, then you'd turn a corner and it's like, presto: the Colosseum!

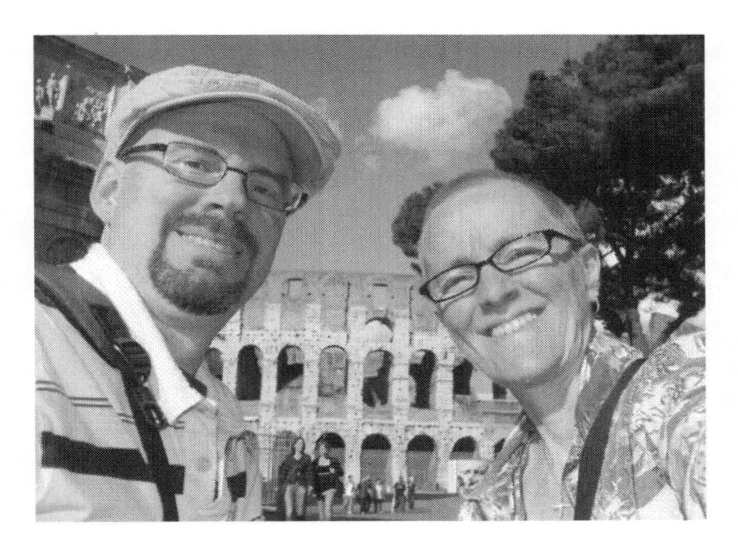

After we toured the Colosseum we sat down on a stone in the Roman Forum to try and catch our breath, which we had checked at the door of the Colosseum. But it was just taken away again when I realized I was sitting in the same place Audrey sat when Gregory Peck found her seemingly drunk and quoting poetry. She wasn't drunk, just "verrrrry haaaappy, not to mention tranquilized." I could relate.

You'd think Dr. Lower had prescribed me gelato the way I took it once or twice a day while I was in Rome. She hadn't. But I wonder if I stumbled onto some kind of alternative medical breakthrough with my gelato binge, I mean, research. Here's what I discovered: I felt a lot better when I was taking gelato regularly. Especially, gelato of the Nutella variety. Now, I'm not the biggest sweet eater in the world, but if you made me eat Nutella gelato every day for the rest of my life I wouldn't hold it against you. The only known side effect of Nutella gelato, besides addiction, which I totally proved (using the scientific method and everything) to be harmless and therefore hardly worth mentioning, is that it can make you do crazy things. Like run up the Spanish Steps and declare your love for Rome and all things Nutella. No, I didn't, actually. I had to pretty much constantly fight the temptation to run like Rocky up those steps—mostly because I was worried the gelato would fall off the sugar cone. I just couldn't risk it.

Audrey didn't go to a tennis match on her Roman holiday, but we did improvise a few things on ours: like the Sistine Chapel, the

Catacombs, and the Rome Masters finals. Just to stay close to the script, though, we rented a Vespa to get to the tennis match.

Rafa—not the port, but the tennis player—was playing in the Rome finals. It was about time the two Rafas met, not on the courts, but at the match. The Rome Masters is a precursor to the French Open and as such, is played on clay, which is Rafa's native surface. I'd always dreamed of watching the King of Clay play on real life clay. Rafa was playing against another one of my favorite players, Novak Djokovic, who'd won the tournament in 2008. It was my best-case scenario finals. Getting to see Rafa vs. Djokovic, was like a tennis fairy tale come true for me. And I will never ever forget the rush of seeing Rafa win on and then wear the red Roman clay. I snapped an awesome victory shot for a memento, but also as a reminder of how I was going to feel when I downed that last chemo cocktail.

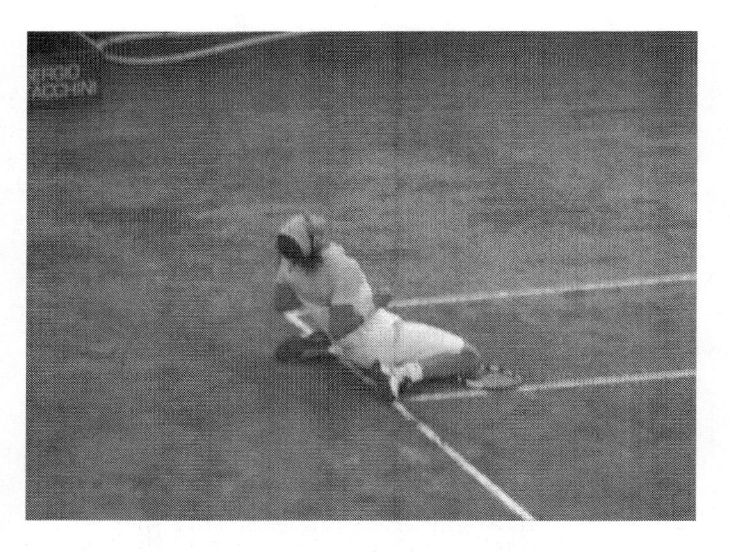

By now you've probably noticed the hole in my Roman holiday plot, and are wondering, "Where's the Mouth of Truth scene?"

Well, it was our last day in Rome and we were tooling around town on the Vespa. We toured the Pantheon. We ordered champagne and cold coffee at a sidewalk café while we discussed the last two things that remained on the list for our Roman holiday: the Mouth of Truth and souvenirs. We still wanted to get a little something for our mums. And I'd been eyeing a Vespa messenger bag all week. Now that I'd been there, done that, I just had to buy the bag.

But first, the Mouth of Truth. In the famous scene, Gregory Peck sticks his hand in the statue's mouth while explaining that legend has it that the statue will bite off the hands of liars. When he pulls out his arm, he has his hand hidden up his jacket sleeve and she didn't have a clue he was going to do that. Her surprise is genuine and so delightfully Audrey.

I couldn't wait to stick my hand in the Mouth of Truth and play the same joke on Dave. Little did I know it wouldn't just bite my hand off, but rather chew me up and spit me out. Or, at least, that's how it felt.

This is the part of the story where the proverbial clock is supposed to strike midnight and I turn into a pumpkin and drive away in my glass slipper. And that will be the end of the fairy tale. Instead, what really happened is that the clock struck three in the afternoon and I was trying to park the Vespa with all the other Vespas parked in front of the Mouth of Truth. I decided it wasn't going to take the hard left I was aiming for, so instead I thought I'd just stop and then walk it over to the spot.

The last thing I remember is Dave yelling, "Brake!" and me thinking, "Duh."

I wasn't braced for impact, because I was squeezing the brake. Not the break. I was just as shocked as Audrey was in her Mouth of Truth scene when all of a sudden I realized my nose was hurting like hell. The Vespa'd hit the wall and I'd followed suit.

I was trailing Dave. He was holding onto the seat upon impact, when he says I disappeared, flew over the handlebars into the wall, and then somehow ended up on the ground underneath the front wheel of the Vespa. It seems I face-planted, which didn't apparently take, since I slid down the wall and underneath the wheel of the Vespa before it fell over, stunned, to the ground. I have no memory of impact but I can't help but picture Wile E. Coyote. Dave can't watch *Road Runner* anymore. Too deja-me. Unfortunately, Port Rafa also hit the wall like a line drive. I was super confused and couldn't figure out why my face and mouth were dripping wet. So I asked Dave to take a picture.

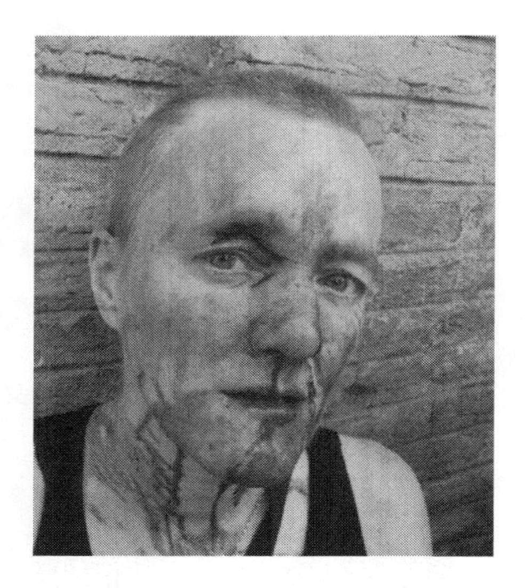

But then I couldn't see it because my glasses were sort of smashed. Dave had a handkerchief and kept applying pressure to try to stop the bleeding until the ambulance came. It freaking hurt and I was trying to remember what happened. I got pretty irritated at him for bugging me about applying pressure, pressure, and more pressure.

I don't remember much of the ambulance ride. In fact, I think I lost the handkerchief there, amidst the rush to get me to the emergency room, where thankfully they practiced the art of being kind to and taking care of strangers. They sewed me back together and stopped the external bleeding. But they had to keep suctioning my nose, because it kept filling up with blood. I kept gagging and felt like I was choking to death because I couldn't breathe, because I was choking on the bleeding that wouldn't stop.

I got five stitches over my right eye and two in my chin. I have no idea how many tests they ran on me: X-rays, a CT scan, an EKG, an ultrasound, and blood tests. They didn't speak much English and I don't speak much Italian, especially not medical Italian. It was scary as hell not knowing what they were doing to me, and I remember being in a state of panic trying to let them know about my port so they wouldn't use my left arm for drawing blood or taking my blood pressure. But I couldn't even think of the word for arm—*braccio*—a lot of good it does me now. And I didn't have a clue what the word for *port* was. They seemed to understand the word *cancer*. And they were kind to me, despite our communication gap. One nurse held my hand. Thank God we had a friend in Rome, Juliet, who came to our rescue, and was able to act as our translator and find out the scoop: a broken nose bone, which was connected to a broken cheekbone, which was connected to a broken jawbone. I don't think it's a mere coincidence that the Italian word for drat is *accidenti*.

After the ER, I was admitted for observation and was taken to a room with three other women. While the nurses transferred me to my bed, a confused, elderly roommate of mine fell out of hers. The nurses quickly ran across the room to help her back into her bed. And then they left the room.

And that is the last time anyone came into our room until around nine-thirty p.m., when a nurse came in and told Dave he had to leave. Visiting hours were over. He couldn't stay in the room since there were three other women in it, and the hospital didn't allow anyone to stay overnight, so he'd have to leave the premises.

There was no way Dave was going to leave me there for observation with no one to watch over me. And there was no way I was going to stay there by myself. We reasoned that it was wiser for Dave to be with me back in the hotel room, than for me to be utterly unattended to in the hospital. I had to have Dave place my hand on the paper I was supposed to sign to get myself out of the hospital. I couldn't actually see the paper I was signing. My glasses were broken and my eyes were practically swollen shut.

We took a taxi back to the B&B. Juliet got some medical supplies, some dinner for Dave, a dish of gelato for me, and then she took care of returning the Vespa to the rental place. Thank God he had an angel there for me in Rome.

We made it to the airport and home safely the next day as scheduled. But. That. Was. THE. Longest night. Of my life. I couldn't breathe. Everything hurt. I couldn't see. I couldn't sleep. All I knew was that Dave desperately needed to get some sleep, because he still had to pack all our things, get us to the airport, then home. All the while keeping me under observation.

Boy was I under observation the whole way home. Dave felt like everybody was looking at him like he did it to me, or something. If I thought people stared at me when I was bald . . . well, that was nothing compared to walking onto a crowded plane with a broken face.

Which sort of brings us back to the beginning, when Audrey is telling the barber to take off all her hair and he says to her, "Your friends, I don't think they will recognize you," to which Princess Anne happily responds, "No, I don't think they will."

I looked so awful that I'm pretty sure the entire plane felt sorry for me. I felt sorry for the children who had to see me. The flight attendants were so kind to me. They were even able to clear an entire middle row of five seats for Dave and me so I could lie down.

I was super worried that my kids were going to freak out if I just walked off the plane looking like that, so I asked Dave to text them a picture of me so it wouldn't be such a shock.

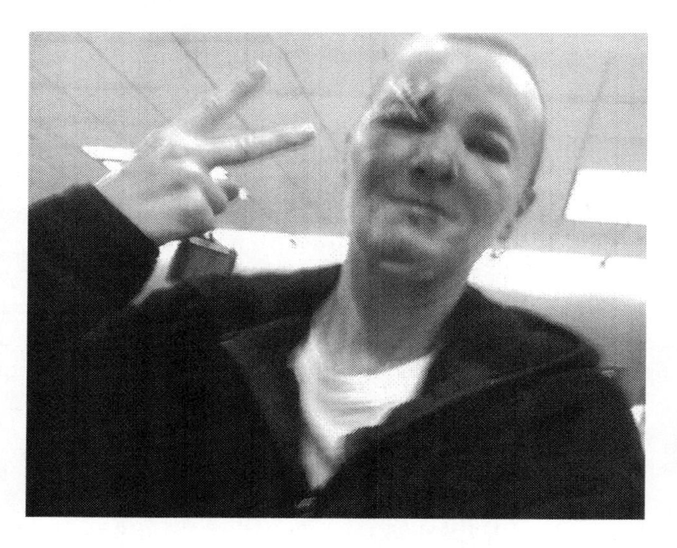

Dave had called them to let them know we'd had a wreck on the Vespa and that I'd been hurt, but he had not told them exactly how badly I was injured, nor how awful I looked. I hadn't gotten to talk to them since the wreck, so Dave put the phone up to my ear and Amanda prayed that God would put all the bones back in place so they wouldn't have to be set again when I got home.

The day after we got back, I had an appointment at the chemo cocktail lounge to down Round 13. I'm not even kidding. I'd purposely planned the trip as far away from Round 12 as possible, with no margin for error, and butting right up into Round 13.

I wasn't feeling amped up for the last twelve chemo cocktails like I'd planned.

I wasn't even sure if my port was going to work for this one. Amazingly, it did.

Dr. Lower was calm and positive, as always, when she asked me about my trip and, by the way, what in the world happened to my face? This both calmed me and excited me, because I couldn't wait to tell her the story.

She must have thought it was a good one, because she suggested I go tell an ENT the story as soon as I finished downing that chemo cocktail. I got an appointment with our ENT on our way home from the chemo cocktail lounge.

Dr. Skurow's exam resulted in yet another—but this time surprisingly hopeful—twist.

"I think you may have dodged a bullet here," he said.

Then he explained that my nose, jaw, and cheekbone were all in place from what he could tell from the manual exam.

I'm not even kidding. Just like Amanda prayed they would be.

Dr. Skurow still had some concern with the cheek, though, and he wanted to see me back in a couple of days, after the swelling went down a little.

Meanwhile, I also saw my dentist to see if he thought my front teeth, which were so numb that I couldn't bite down on anything, were going to completely lose their nerve and fall out. My dentist referred me to an oral-facial surgeon who took a bunch of Star Trekky pictures of the structure of what was beginning to resemble the outline of my face.

Then I went back to Dr. Skurow's so he could check my cheek. He took out my stitches and what felt like my right eyelid with them. He also ordered a CT scan to verify that the structure of my right eye was sound. And then he referred me to an ophthalmologist for further specialized examination and explanation.

The consensus of all the aforementioned doctors was that I had a depressed orbit. Which, when I've tried to put myself in that eye socket's place, seems to be perfectly understandable, considering all it had gone through. The good news was that the orbit floor of my right eye was not a blowout fracture, which everyone was worried about, since the orbit floor is a tissue-thin bone that supports the eyeball and keeps it from falling into the sinus cavity. I'd actually lapped worry and was in a constant state of panic over the thought of blowing my eyeball out my nose. And I'd been blowing my nose like crazy. But thankfully, even though the orbit floor was broken, it was still intact, even if it was depressed. Probably the only time in the history of the world a depressed eye orbit was a slightly cheerful diagnosis.

The ophthalmologist basically told me we'd just keep a proverbial "eye" on things, let me heal, and to call if I experienced any double vision. Double vision could be a sign of my eye muscles getting snagged on bone fragments from the fracture. Also he told me not to blow my nose until further notice. Other than that, I asked him if I could play tennis and he said yes, which was pretty much like saying "Cheers!" to me.

Now, onto cheering up that depressed orbit.

Rounds 14 and 15
Backwards

When you just read the title for this chapter, you probably thought, "Now what?" And I went back and forth about whether to go ahead and let you think that for awhile, or if I should [*spoiler alert*] put to rest any fears of more crap happening to me.

I thought about tossing a coin to decide, but in the end I tossed the coin aside (it was heads, if you were wondering) and decided instead, to take a chance with you, gentle reader. You see, as I typed B-A-C-K-W-A-R-D-S (and no, I don't have the superpower of literally typing words backwards, unlike those servers who write their names upside down on the tablecloth when they hand you a menu and take down your drink order), I had a sympathy pain for you shoot straight into my heart. I cringed when I imagined you turning the page and reading that word *Backwards* at the top of the page. (And by backwards, *I know you know what I mean.* Seriously, if we keep going off on silly tangents like that we are never going to get to the happy ending part of the story. After all, I promised you a comedy about my tragedy. So let's just put all those nasty twists of my fate behind us and move forward, channeling our inner rhinos now, shall we?)[42]

Anyway, as I was saying, I know your first thought after reading that word was one of sheer panic for me, the *I* in this memoir, because you're super thoughtful like that. I can just tell. And I realize the way things have been going up to this point you were probably *expecting* the proverbial other shoe to drop. From the sky. With me in it. Or under it. Or something like that.

And I simply couldn't do that to you. Even at the risk of you possibly thinking that this chapter might get a little boring without all the drama, and deciding to skip ahead to the comedy part. By the way, it's on page 225 See, I just went ahead and showed my hand. *That's* how much I trust you not to leave me hanging. Plus, this *is* a memoir, and I *am* trying to be vulnerable here. Even if it is hard for me, because I'm shyer than, coincidentally, a Sumatran rhinoceros.

The thing is, when I was sitting out on the back porch gathering up my backstory for the writing of this here chapter, I had the song "Backwards" by Rascal Flatts playing in the background. On loop. And once the story started humming along it was one step forward and two-stepping it backwards all the way.

Just like the song, which is based on the old joke, "What do you get when you play country music backwards?" Well, my first verse is: I got my hair back. Not all of it, and not all at once. But you've read the "Wind in My Hair" chapter, so I'm not telling you something you don't already know. But there's more.

It was finally summer, so I got my back deck back. Now, I know the song says front porch swing, not back deck. I'm not trying to ruin the song for all you front porch swing lovers. It's just that I don't have a front porch swing. I barely have a front porch. But, I have a back deck. To me, it serves a similar function, minus the swinging part, of course. Especially since it overlooks the tennis courts behind my house. Sometimes if my friends have a dispute over whether or not a ball was in, they call up to me and I make the official line call for them. I know I could probably put my kids through college by charging for this neighborly service, on top of writing off my sunroom as a business expense. But at the moment I already had two full-time jobs with teaching and fighting cancer. It wasn't the right time for a career change.

Getting my back deck back meant getting summer back. I was made for summer. Last fall when my hair fell, and then the chemo scared it into hibernation for the winter, there were days I couldn't see as far as a bad hair day in the spring, let alone a gentle breeze playing with my hair on my back deck in the summer. And yet, there I was. After Round 14, I must have been enjoying myself so much that I actually forgot to blog about it. I didn't even mention it.

There's just a gap that I probably spent sitting on my back deck being gloriously boring.

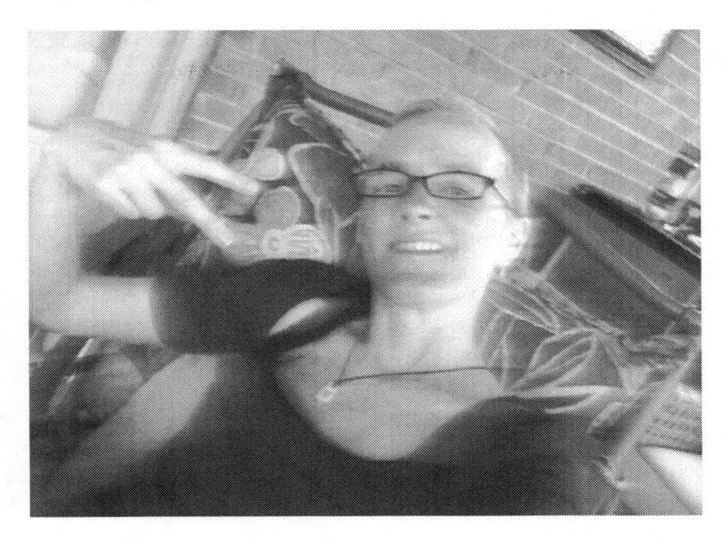

Getting summer back also meant that we actually made it through the most challenging homeschool and co-op year *ever*. Despite the craziness, I'm quite proud of what we accomplished. I don't know what I would've done if Mikeyy hadn't met some of the students from the co-op and asked me if we could join it, because there is no way we could've made it through this year without a little help from our friends. It also helped me with my own homeschool planning. In our homeschool I'd always integrated history with literature and composition, which is usually what I spent the bulk of my summer working on. Since I was cross-teaching the literature part with my Brit Lit class, and had to mail my students a syllabus and book list shortly after summer break began, I had lots of extra motivators during my lesson planning. Fifteen extra motivators—and their parents. I was so glad that I had the entire year penciled-in on my school planner, down to how many pages I expected them to read a day, before the cancer hit. I had to keep up with the reading to lead class discussion and grade and dialogue with the daily reading journals I had them keep, which was the hard part during the hardest part of chemo because the fog was thick to read through. But I managed somehow. Not only that, I really think that focusing so hard on managing that course load was therapeutic in my own cancer battle because it took my mind off the chemo. Fifteen delightful distractions. Also I kept remembering Linda had been there and done that for my Mikeyy, and it inspired me to pay it forward.

With the summer breeze, I was also beginning to feel like my mind was back for the most part, since the chemo fog had pretty much lifted. The shape of it was debatable; sure, I'll admit it. Between the fallout from chemo brain and the collateral damage from the Vespa incident, there were plenty of reasons to worry about my brain bouncing back.

My nerves, on the other hand, were still a wreck from the wreck. After Round 14, apparently the most boring chemo cocktail round in my history, Dr. Skurow had given me the thumbs up on the healing process concerning my broken face. But my front upper right teeth were still numb and felt a little loose. I had to knife and fork everything into tiny bites, and then chew way back on the left side of my mouth, which was a pain. Not in the painful sense, though. My teeth didn't actually hurt. They just felt like they might not hold fast, which made me nervous. But that was a whole different ball of nerves. My jaw was still sore from the jar it took, which added to the chewing issues. Plus it was tiring and slightly painful if I got in a chatty mood. My forehead and the tips of my nose and chinny-chin-chin were still numb, and Dr. Skurow said those sensory nerves would be the last things to heal. So I was trying not to let them get on my nerves. It helped when Dr. Skurow reminded me how lucky I was, and that if I had to crash, I did it right. Got my pride back a little, too.

One of the things that made me so proud I almost imploded was watching Amanda try out for *American Idol* in Chicago. She didn't sing a country song backwards or anything. She sang a little Sixpence, and I about kissed her the way she showed me how it's done when you don't let anything hold you back from chasing your dreams. She didn't let not moving forward to the next round of auditions keep her from forming a band and cutting her first CD. On top of that, she called me out on one of my own dreams, while I was sitting at my laptop posting an update for her fans back home. "Mum, once you get your health back I think you should chase your own dream and turn that blog into a book . . . Yep, it's gonna happen. You're going to do it."

Yep, I got my own advice back.

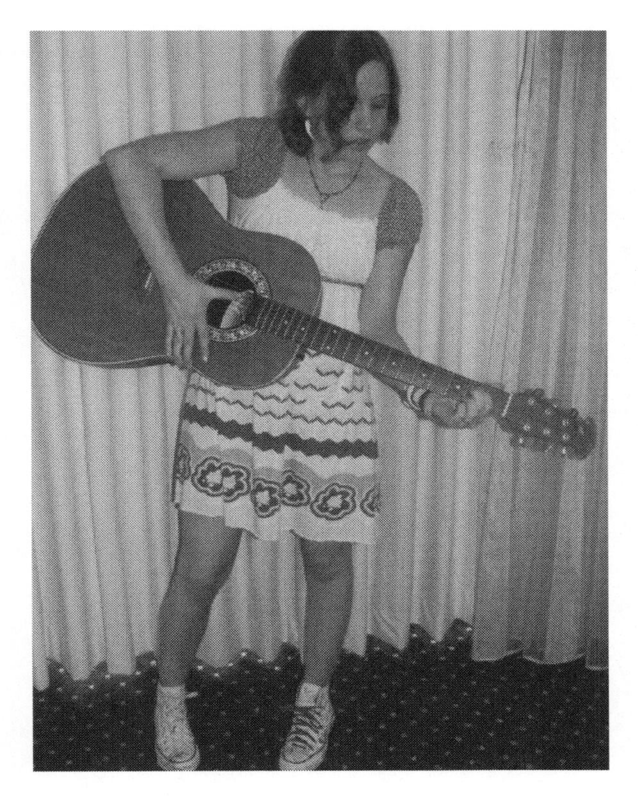

I also got tennis back. Quite a lot of tennis since it was summer. One of my tennis girlfriends told me I was about fifty-five to sixty percent back. I'm not saying it was pretty tennis or anything, but it felt like Christmas in June to me, to be out there again. I even had a sock tan going, which is a super sexy thing in the tennis world, if you didn't already know. I had to improvise a new serve because of the port, which was a bit of a powder-puff serve, but at least I could put a ball in play. And once I was in a point, I was able to keep up with it. I didn't have my strength, stamina, or speed quite back, but I was getting there. I could feel myself getting stronger and faster, despite my neuropathetic feet, which sometimes felt like cement blocks. I kept thinking that if I kept pounding the courts with them, the blood would keep circulating, and eventually pay the Tax-ALL bill.

I played my first USTA match. It was doubles, and my partner and I WON! In two sets! So. Good. To be back.

And I know that playing country music backwards has nothing to do with playing tennis, but when it says something about getting your life back—well, for me, tennis was a big part. Things were turning around.

After I downed Round 15, I could count my remaining chemo cocktails on two hands. It was time to begin counting backwards. T minus ten, the countdown, would be ready to commence in three weeks.

---

[42] Some legends have it that rhinos can't walk backwards. It's my story, after all, and I'm sticking to it.

Rounds 16 and 17
I'm on a Roll

It had been ten months since Dr. Stahl had removed the damn spots, and it was time for a checkup. I'm supposed to see her every six months, and was supposed to check in right after we got back from Rome. But I had so many emergency doctor's appointments trying to put my Humpty Dumpty face back together that something had to give. All the little boxes on my calendar were so optimistic that they were spilling over, blurring the lines between the days of my life. Somehow, my checkup rolled down that slippery slope and fell through a crack in the calendar, where we found it two months later. Time really does fly when you're on a roll like that.

I think I was sitting in the ophthalmologist's office, waiting to hear if he thought my poor eye was going to do one of those meatball-on-top-of-spaghetti tricks the next time I sneezed, when I realized that, as long as my eyeball was still intact, I couldn't possibly be in both doctor's offices at once. Regretfully, I called Dr. Stahl's office to reschedule. And thankfully, the ophthalmologist simply told me not to sneeze, or no gesundheit for me. Any future rolling of my eyes from now on would be nothing more than a response to one of Dave's jokes.

I was a bit nervous going in for the checkup. I didn't want anything to rain on my parade, if you know what I mean. Not that I have anything against singing in the rain, or umbrellas, for that matter. Especially if there are polka dots on the umbrella, which I think cheer up almost any dreary day. That's really all I know to do when it rains. Either that, or stay inside and make grilled cheese sandwiches and tomato soup. And if you toss in some colorful goldfish crackers, you get the same polka dot effect. Plus it takes your mind off the storm, to focus on fishing for goldfish in your tomato soup.

But I was trying to channel my inner Annie and hope for the sun to come out and play.

Plus, the truth is, I couldn't wait to tell Rita about Port Rafa and the Vespa incident. Telling the story was the one perk I extrapolated from the Vespa incident. I figure if you have to go through something like that, you oughta at least be able to salvage a good story out of it. Rita had been so kind to field all my phone calls, queries, and complaints about my port and the pain in my pec, so I owed her a good story. For all those trying times, like when I peppered her with questions about if it was really and truly positively without a doubt OK to play competitive tennis because what if I took a tennis ball to the port? Would it, could it, damage or dislodge it? She said it would take a really hard line drive with a baseball or something harder than that. Boy, did I have a good one.

I knew she wasn't expecting *me* to take a line drive at a Roman wall to prove her theory, but I thought she'd appreciate the you-were-right confession from me. Which she did, and not in that rub-your-nose-in-it kind of way. I mean, who doesn't mind a little vindication now and then?

Besides the good story, I got a very good report that day. Basically Dr. Stahl broke down her exam like this for me: she was looking for peas in the pod, but didn't find any. In other words, I passed the exam. In tennis terms, you might say I aced it.

I loved it when she said there were no peas in the pod. I didn't mind that she compared it to peas, because there weren't any, and also I thought it was super cool that my breast surgeon spoke in code like that. It took me back to my secret agent training days. But it also was a doctor vindicating, as it were, my own personal distaste of peas, for eating purposes. They are perfectly good choices for an ice pack in a pinch. Case in point, when Amanda and Mikeyy had their wisdom teeth extracted at the same time. I had ice packs for them and everything, but if I hadn't, I totally would have borrowed a few bags of peas from my neighbors.

Other than that, I have no use for peas. Although I do have to admit that I do love those hilarious French Peas on *VeggieTales*. But not in the way that it would make me want to clean my plate if there was a mound of peas, not even adorable slushie-throwing French ones, taunting me.

Note that I did not say side dish, because I would never serve up a side dish of peas, since I figure the golden rule applies in the reciprocal. As a side note, it felt like home again to have the roles reversed, where I was just another mum feeding her poor chipmunk-cheeked children a steady diet of ice cream and copious amounts of TLC.

The chemo cocktail countdown continued a couple of days after the checkup. I couldn't wait to put Round 16 in the wake of chemo cocktails behind me. The anticipation of being done with cancer was increasing as I counted down. Momentum was on my side. I was on a roll. I could say it was like a snowball effect, but I don't really enjoy the cold, so I don't feel like going there—*brrrr*. Anyway, "I'm on a roll," says a whole lot more, with less, when you really think about it.

Speaking of cold, Dr. Lower ran a blood test before commencing T minus nine, to check on my thyroid because my thermostat was having some issues. It was probably just a side effect of the chemo, but she wanted to establish a baseline to keep an eye on it in case it didn't chill out. Previously, my dial only read cold, goosebumps, teeth chattering, and somewhere in between defrost and thaw. Chemo had added melt to the mix while simultaneously mixing the signals from head to toe. My face would be melting off. I'd have goosebumps all over my arms that I couldn't seem to warm with my hot and sweaty hands. And my feet would be cold and clammy like blocks of ice. The blood test came back fine. My thyroid was just off somewhere, trying to find its groove. Just like I'd found my new chemo cocktail groove with each new mix.

By the time T minus nine went down, I was pretty much a Herceptin-only expert. Dave must have gotten bored or something, because he calculated how many drops of Herceptin I would get during the ninety-minute drip: 4,320. It's possible he counted them one by one. Like sands through the hourglass—no, I wasn't watching soap operas while he crunched the numbers.

We watched Food Network in the chemo cocktail lounge. As usual I was imagining that the TV was my video menu, so I was trying to figure out what I was in the mood for on a T minus nine kind of day.

That day I was seated next to the elder sisters. They were two sisters who always came together (one was hooked up to a chemo cocktail like me; the second was her sidekick, like Dave). They were usually delightfully chatty, which I always enjoyed, because it's not like I could keep up counting the drips drop like Dave. They liked watching Food Network too, and provided hilarious commentary while we watched.

During one commercial, they had a little sidebar conversation about me liking to cook. I was still sitting there, with them. We were sharing a TV tray. I hadn't left the room or even my lounge chair. I looked up at my IV, which I never got brave enough to drag around no matter how badly I had to pee from all the liquids drip-drip-dripping, and I was still attached to it. We were all sitting in a row of recliners in front of the same TV. So I wasn't exactly eavesdropping when I overheard the one with the IV say, and I quote, "You can't really trust a skinny cook."

Totally caught me off guard. I almost broke my face again trying to keep from cracking up while I butted in of course, in my own defense.

"But I use butter! Lots and lots of butter. Real butter. There is Julia, Julie, and Joules. We're practically three of a kind when it comes to butter. Also, I use whole milk. And heavy cream. I'd also like to point out the fact that I just say no to anything that says lite or non-fat." I thought I'd offered an airtight defense. She gave me props, but I could tell she was still nursing a kernel of suspicion with her chemo cocktail.

I have to be honest. I felt like the case was closed and that I'd been vindicated when the other sister changed the subject to her sister's brand new digital hi-def TVs. Apparently, she'd bought two of them in successive unsuccessful efforts to replace her old one and was super frustrated because she could still only get two or three channels on any given TV. But the sans-IV sister said the real problem was that IV sister was too stubborn to ante up for cable.

Seems like the frustration erupted eventually because sans-IV sister said that, at one point, IV sister called her and before she could get the phone up to her ear she heard, "The instructions say something about a cursor. What the hell is a cursor?!" Then, silence. At which point sans-IV sister thought it was safe to bring the phone back up to her ear. Just in time to hear, "Oh . . . I guess I am."

It was chemo cocktail lounge entertainment at its finest.

A lot of the time the other patrons are sleeping, or chatting with their lounge dates, or reading, Sudokuing, or texting or talking on cell phones, so it's not always that exciting in the chemo cocktail lounge.

Sometimes there were very sick patients right next to me and it sort of broke my heart. I know we were both sitting there in identical pale green recliners hooked up to IVs that look similar, except for the name, birthdate, and Rx on the bags. But still, there was a part of me that kept forgetting I was fighting for my life—until the quiet man next to me would ask for some ice chips because he can't eat, because he has a feeding tube. Or the woman across the room from me whose port wouldn't work anymore. She said she had tried everything and was just about to stand on her head if this next poke didn't work. Or the frail woman next to me who had to be unhooked and taken to the hospital by ambulance because she had pneumonia.

There's always a reality check underneath it all. Always something to snap me out of it, to remind me not to let myself go home and waste the next three weeks, because they are a gift. Just like the health and fitness I was rebuilding. I was on a roll. Sixteen chemo cocktails down, and counting.

Before commencing countdown at T minus eight, I had another MUGA scan. It had been three months since my last round of radioactivity. Got the same old normal report back. Which is curious, when you think about scans that come back normal when there are radioactive tracers surging throughout my body. Hmm.

Here's a snapshot from one typical radioactive day in my life.

First I woke up, at approximately the butt crack of dawn, to go to the hospital and get my radioactive shot. I have to schedule my MUGA scans early since I'm not allowed to have anything to eat or drink until after I'm radioactive. Which includes coffee. Which doesn't make sense to me, because the last thing I'd think the hospital staff would want on their consciences is a decaffeinated superhero. And especially not a cranky one.

Anyway, next, I drove home to pick up Matt, who jumped in the car. He had to, because I wasn't stopping till we got to the coffee shop to get my fix, I mean, so he could meet a friend.

Then I went to the bank for Amanda and stopped off to get a carrot juice at Aladdin's Eatery, a cute little Mediterranean bistro I frequent so often they think I'm one of the busboys. (I guess it's the hairdo.) And yeah, that's what superheroes drink. I dare you to try it.

Then I went home and took a **SUPERPOWER NAP**, after which I awoke in the nick of time to pick up Mikeyy from a film camp he was attending that week.

I hope it didn't come off too boastful, me telling you about my supernapping power in bold and all caps like that. I wasn't trying to yell it at the top of my lungs and get you in trouble if you happen to be sitting in the library or something. It's just that it didn't look right leaving *superpower nap* in normal type. It wasn't just any nap. And I didn't take it for granted one bit. The coolest thing about it was at the end of the day, I'd been able to do one small thing for each of my kids, which was in part fueled by that awesome nap. Which is why I don't mind admitting that I heart naps. Because at the end of the day, all I really want to be is Supermum with a capital *S* (a red one) to my kids.

Evidently I had some residual radioactivity left when I went in for Round 17, because as we commenced T minus eight, I decided to recline my chemo lounger and accidentally pulled the handle right off. First I felt cool. Then I felt bad for breaking the chair. And when I came to my senses quite a few hours later, I felt a tad bit careless, that I'd almost blown my own cover.

Luckily, most of the potential witnesses were distracted by the new flatscreen TV in the chemo lounge. Thank God for technology.

Still, this presented quite a predicament for Dave, who hasn't met a button that he isn't dying to push. When he's not counting the drips on my IV, Dave's favorite pastime is adjusting the proper screen ratio and whatnot on a widescreen. We do not buy full screen movies in the Evanshire. We just don't go there, for Dave's sake. It's a misnomer he can't abide. When there is only sixty-six percent of the movie on the screen, there really is no optimizing that can possibly make him happy.

I practically read his mind before he even knew what he was thinking, so I knew exactly what he was going to say, even before he tugged at his mustache like he does, and said, "Doesn't it bother you the way it's all stretched out on the screen?"

"We don't have the remote," I countered. It was sitting on a TV tray, which was underneath the TV. Across the room from us. Out of reach. Checkmate. I was hooked up to an IV and stuck in my lounger, and honestly, I wasn't in the mood to be bothered by the fact that the French fries Rachael Ray was making were not proportional. What is a proper portion of French fries, anyway? And who *doesn't* want more than their fair share when it comes to French fries? I didn't really see his point. Besides that, he was also sitting in a recliner, which obviously meant he wasn't going to be getting up anytime soon. Not even to push a button.

Luckily, there was a newspaper that some kind soul had left in the lounge, sitting on the tray between us. I thought quickly, turned to the crossword section, and successfully diverted his attention from the dilemma at hand. There were two crosswords, one easy and one advanced. I'm still trying to process what it means that we finished the advanced puzzle in half the time it took us to solve the easy one.

Somewhere in the middle of our crossword puzzles, a woman across the room from us asked one of the nurses for a single malt to be hooked into her IV. Her nurse didn't catch the reference, so I said, "She wants a Scotch." Which was the wrong thing to say, because then all Dave could think about was opening up a bar in the chemo lounge.

Interestingly, there was a woman there, with her husband, getting the tour from Dr. Lower's nurse. It was her first chemo. I remembered that tour. Also, there was another woman there, receiving her last chemo. I totally high-fived her as I left the chemo lounge. It was so surreal sitting there, with my past in a room behind me, and my future in the next chair.

Seventeen down, seven up. I was so on a roll.

Round 18
Lucky Star

Perseus didn't shower and the stars weren't blue when my calendar had traveled a full orbit, displaying August 11 once again. I felt like I should commemorate that august night, and by all means celebrate the fact that I'd taken a whole trip around the sun since Mikeyy and I had been lucky enough to take in the meteor show the night before our world was shaken. I didn't read my horoscope the morning of eight-eleven. I didn't play connect the dots or try to find a message in the stars that night. I knew they were up there, twinkle-twinkling, but I didn't have to wonder. I knew they were my lucky stars. I was the luckiest girl in the world, by far.

It was obvious, to me at least: Somebody out there loved me, and that was good enough for me.

I spent the day with my boys, taking them school shopping. I've always loved taking the kids school supply shopping. They, however, do not share my enthusiasm for getting new pencils and cool notebooks. But they have, at least, always indulged me. They are sweet like that. Mikeyy even let himself act a little excited with me over the new Zebra mechanical pencils we discovered, which meant a lot to this pencil (I heart pencils) pusher. Especially since, as it was to be our final year of homeschooling, it would also be the last home school supply shopping field trip *ever*.

That evening I went out with a few girlfriends from the homeschool co-op. We went to see *Julie & Julia.* I ordered a large popcorn with butter—it seemed wrong not to. Of course I shared it. Popcorn is made for sharing. Especially when you're out with a bunch of homeschool mums, who seem to get as much fun out of divvying up the popcorn into equal portions as they do eating it—all the while discussing art projects with popcorn, the myth of popcorn at the first Thanksgiving, and science fair projects on how popcorn pops. The hard part is keeping them from multitasking while they watch the movie. When they break out the needle and thread and start stringing the popcorn, that's when I think it's time for a little time out.

After the movie, we debriefed over fish tacos at Mitchell's Fish Market on the Levee. We wined and dined outdoors, overlooking the Ohio River, and underneath the night sky, where the archer was aiming at the scorpion. I don't know what the scorpion ever did to him, but I sure wish the archer would take out that damn crab instead.

These homeschool mums were a vital part of my cancer fighting team. They prayed over me before I left the co-op every single chemo Monday. Which is what I like to call perfect attendance. They prayed over me like mothers pray, and I believed like a child. They had compassion on me and encouraged me. It was a little like I was Frodo and they were the Fellowship. It was fitting, then, to break bread and drink wine with them to celebrate how we'd gone there and back again. Then they prayed over me that night, before I went home.

When I got home I chased the wine with an Ativan and tried to count sheep to keep my mind off marbles. But, every time I'd start to drift off, Sagittarius would shoot one of the sheep. I kept losing track counting and would have to start over, again and again. I know the poor sheep must've been exhausted with all that jumping back and forth over fences while I tried to get an accurate count. I never did. Eventually the sandman was called in, the sheep got some rest, and I got a better night's sleep than I had a year ago that night. No marbles haunted my dreams.

That anniversary was the first domino to fall, in a line of cancerversaries. If you know me, you know there was no lumping them all together like some sort of cancer collage. Each cancerversary required its own frame. I admit that I'm a control freak with OCD *leanings.* (In fact, I even specifically chose the word leanings, then *italicized* it to **emphasize** it. Not only that, I can't even tell you how happy it made me to slam down that italicize-emphasize rhyme.) Anyway, I guess I've pretty much always had a little OCD though I don't know why people have to go calling it a disorder. Just because, for instance, I'm not a fan of the old *heaping helping* method of plating food to the point that it overlaps. It simply overwhelms me and sort of confuses me. I mean, wouldn't it be more accurate to label messy plates with disorder? Now, please note: I don't mean to point any fingers at people who pile food on my plate. Au contraire, mon ami! Pointing is rude and I don't feel like being rude to people, especially people who feed me. Thanks to being a grown up and also that spy training, I've gotten pretty skilled at doing damage control with subtle fork action and some distracting chitchat. The hand being faster than the eye, so to speak. When I was a kid I used to separate candy corn with a knife, then collate all the pieces into three neat piles. First I'd eat the yellow pieces, then the orange ones, and I'd save the white tips for last. They were my favorite and it felt so unfair that they made up such a small fraction of the candy corn, which really was more like a cone, if you ask me. And the thing is, if they'd have called it candy cone instead, then inverted it, of course, it would've totally made sense for the white to be the á la mode as it were. But they didn't. As it was, if only they would've made the white part the base, I would've been spared quite a lot of Halloween stress as a kid. Now I've learned to eat them whole, and by the handful. But every once in a while I'll just eat the white parts off a handful of candy corn, for nostalgia's sake. I wonder why I didn't think of that when I was a kid?

Anyway, all that to say, I may still be a tad childish when it comes to celebrating milestones, like anniversaries and counting down chemo cocktails. But I have to be; otherwise, I lose track of my progress like I do when I'm counting sheep.

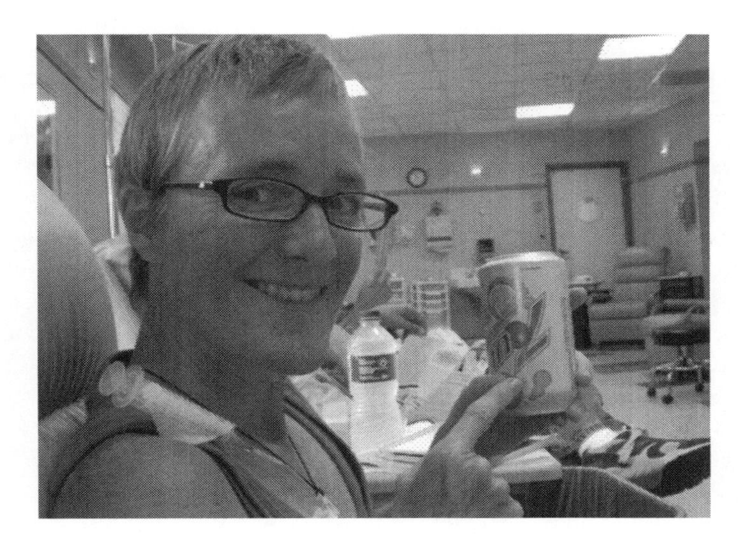

I bought a can of 7UP to commemorate T minus seven, Round 18. I didn't mix it in the chemo cocktail though. For one, it was diet. I don't know if the 7UP man was snoozing on the job when he filled the machine, or if I got distracted trying to flatten out the dollar bill so the machine would accept it and accidentally pushed the wrong button. It remains a mystery to this day. The other reason I didn't drink the 7UP was that I really just bought it to take a picture of me holding the can and pointing to the *7*, which was upside down. I held it upside down on purpose, to illustrate of course that I had downed T minus seven. Which was another reason I didn't open the can, because I probably would've gotten in trouble for making a mess in the chemo lounge. Generally I don't try to get in trouble. Generally I don't have to try.

While I was taking the photo and talking about having only six chemo cocktails left, a guy sitting next to me named Andy, who had on a black bracelet that said Fuck Cancer (which I'd been admiring), gave me a fist pump and said congrats. Then he said he wished he knew how many more he had. I asked him to tell me his story and he told me he had pancreatic cancer and is on chemo until it doesn't work anymore. Which broke my heart. I wanted to drink something, to his health, right then. But not Diet 7UP.

I'd seen Andy from across the room a few times before, but he was usually sleeping. When I walked into the chemo lounge and saw him awake that time, I sat next to him on purpose, and I'm so glad I did. Now he was more than a face across the room that I prayed for without knowing his name. Now he was my friend Andy with the Fuck Cancer bracelet, whom I would look forward to hanging out with at the chemo cocktail lounge.

As soon as we got home from Round 18, we packed Yukon for a family road trip to celebrate my cancerversary milestones, literally, as in, on the road. Dave had a business trip to D.C. and we were tagging along to squeeze in a bit of a holiday before school started up again. My chemo/Vespa incident doctor schedule was a bit of a calendar hog. It even ate up the boys' spring break, and I felt bad about it. Like they say, a doctor a day keeps the apples away . . . no wait, that's not right exactly. No, it wasn't right at all. And we weren't going to miss a perfect opportunity of mixing a little pleasure with Dave's business. In fact, we decided, why not take a bite out of the Big Apple "on our way home." I know you probably ran and just got a map because you're thinking, "Hey, NYC is not exactly on the way home from D.C. to OH." All I can tell you is that when I'm navigating, it can happen.

I hit a second major milestone while we were in D.C. August 20 was the anniversary of the day my breast surgeon said the *C* word to me, and probably the most earth-shaking day of my life. If this were a novel, it would be what I'd call our protagonist's inciting incident. So taking another trip around the sun while the aftershock calmed begged for a little resolution. We didn't go to Disneyland. We spent the day at the Smithsonian, touring the exhibits from *Night at the Museum*. We weren't the only ones standing in line to take pictures giving dum-dum some gum. My blog was short and sweet that day:

> A year ago today . . . I got a lumpectomy that turned out to be cancer. Today I'm going to the Smithsonian with M&M. This is way more fun.

The Big Apple was delicious. So was the pizza. Matt took us on a Spider-Man tour that was one of the most fun literary tours I've ever been on. The crazy part was, he'd never been to New York City before, unless you count swinging from the skyscrapers and battling supervillains on his Xbox 360 Spider-Man games. He showed us Peter Parker's apartment, Doc Ock's lab, Joe's Pizza (the pizza parlor Peter Parker got fired from—coincidentally, my hubby asked the manager why in the world he fired Spider-Man, and he said, matter of factly that he kept showing up late) and finally, the *Daily Bugle* (where

Peter Parker worked). Along the way, my son the tour guide pointed out various buildings telling us both the names of the buildings and the villains he defeated on each of them. It was uncanny how he knew his way around. By the time we climbed the Empire State Building, it had been an affair I will always remember. I was smitten. Been there, done that, bought my own I Heart NY T-shirt.

New York City summed up my year of cancer like I couldn't: from ground zero to the top of the world, where I could practically high-five my lucky stars.

Round 19
Whip It Good

There were a couple more dominos to fall once we got back from New York City. August 29 was the anniversary of my mastectomy. It probably doesn't shock anyone that the first thing that popped into my head was, "Let's throw a party!" I couldn't wait. It had been one hell of a year, having my boobs cut off, downing chemo cocktails, losing my hair, and of course the Vespa incident. It felt surreal, in an incredible sort of a way, to be standing there. Putting the old notch in my cancer ass-kicking belt felt intoxicating! And everyone knows that you're not supposed to be intoxicated alone. I mean, where would the fun be in that? In other words, now that I had hair, I felt like it was time to let it down a little.

I'd buy the flowers (just like Mrs. Dalloway) and the wine (this would be a not-a-chemo-cocktail party). I'd prepare the food (as opposed to the amazing bedside table service I'd received over the past year). And I'd invite all my friends, who'd pretty much walked through hell and back with me that year. I'd thank them all profusely, knowing that it would feel so inadequate. We'd eat, drink, and make merry. I'd just pour generously, and hope Jesus could take my gratitude and do something with it, like when he turned water into wine.[43]

There was just one kink in my plan. The twenty-ninth wasn't working for anybody but me. Yeah, part of me thought, "Fine time for the world to stop spinning around me." But most of me figured everybody could probably use a little breather from all the drama those damn spots had caused.

Dave was away on a business trip that kept extending. He didn't know if he would be able to wrap things up to be home for a party on *the* day, and he didn't want to disappoint me. Um . . . too late.

It's possible that I didn't respond with what might be misconstrued as patience and understanding when he asked if I minded moving the party back and having it on another day. Oh, I'm afraid he construed me, all right. Poor guy.

It was like the helium in my happy, party-planning, balloon-filled thoughts fizzled and deflated, and then all the balloons sunk to the ground. Where they popped. And made a surprisingly ugly mess, for what only a second ago was a big bouquet of beautiful balloons that could float a house all the way to wherever *Up* is. It's not like Dave was caught off guard, seeing balloons popping all over the place. He knows that, for me, not celebrating on *the* day is like waking up, sniffing the coffee, and only being able to find the decaf that you keep on hand for company. I mean, I love my friends and all, but I don't get the point of decaf, any more than I get the idea of a virgin Cosmopolitan. Decaf is like when you pour salt on air-popped popcorn—it just doesn't stick.

Amanda's work schedule was also raining on my parade. Not that she could help it, any more than Dave could help using up all his vacation days taking me to doctor's appointments, surgeries, and chemo. Saturdays were Amanda's busiest days. First, she did nails at the Mandarine Spa all day, then she was a noodle ambassador at Noodles & Company, till closing. Once upon a time there was a nail tech with prunes instead of fingers, and she couldn't seem to keep her own nails polished. That poor nail tech was Amanda. Sad but true story. She was too new at the salon to ask off, and she couldn't find a sub for her shift at Noodles.

Mikeyy was on the tech team at church and it was his weekend to run the soundboard for the high school services.

Matt was the only one who was available. He had the weekend off from playing guitar in the high school worship band.

Kind of hard to plan a party when three out of four of your own family members have already given you their regrets, before you've even thought about buying the vodka to spike the punch with. Tic-tac-toe, party's over. Or three strikes in a row, it's over and out. And boy, could you use that vodka about now.

Plan B was just as shaky. It was really hard to plan anything at all, since I didn't know when Dave was going to be home. Talk about throwing a monkey wrench into my party plans. So we scaled back and made a tentative Plan B with our friends Bob and Debbie. If Dave got back in town, we'd double date and share Spanish wine and tapas.

It was tragic, finding out how many of my friends didn't even know what tapas were. When everyone kept asking how I planned on celebrating, and I told them, I can't even tell you how many times I got this response: "You're going to a *topless* restaurant on the anniversary of your mastectomy? That's . . . um, *bold.*"

Um, no.

I thought it might get old dealing with such an epic misunderstanding, over and over again, spelling out T-A-P-A-S like I was in some sort of a spelling bee, followed by endless lessons on the art and sophistication of T-A-P-A-S wining (did I mention the Sangria?) and dining. But it didn't really. The faces people made when they thought they heard *topless* alone made it worth it. I actually enjoyed every minute of it as a sort of a consolation prize for not getting to have the world revolve around me and my party.

Plan C was more of a pity party, which involved me getting loopy, and Lesley Gore looping on my iPod.[44]

Enter the hero: Matt aka The Mastermind. Matt, especially, was not a fan of potential Plan C, since he'd be the one stuck at home with such a big, fat crybaby. Now, normally Matt's a super laid-back, gamer kind of a guy. But when his Spidey sense sensed the possibility of my dreaded Plan C, putting a kink in the swinging-from-skyscrapers-in-the-Big-Apple-fighting-bad-guys kind of an evening he'd planned, he decided Plan C was a far worse potential nemesis than the Green Goblin and Doctor Octopus combined. So, he called Mr. Incredible, which is, to say, his Daddy-O, and together they staged a coup de my surprise-party plan. On Wednesday. The party was to be on Saturday. Even though Dave was still just a *maybe* at that point, he thought he was going to be able to swing it. Not that they let me in on this development. Nope. They just let me mope like a dope, all week long. Oh, the tangled web of deceit Matt had begun to spin.

First, Spider-Matt roped in his siblings, who both secretly *were* able to get the night off. Then the trio made a secret Facebook event and enlisted the help of a few friends to extend the invite. Then they coordinated everything from my Happy One-Year Cancer-Free cake, to a mix of my chemo cocktail music, to having everyone park in the tennis parking lot behind the Evanshire so I wouldn't see the cars—or the surprise—coming.

Eventually I was given a certain level of clearance. Matt didn't want to take any chances of me letting my ears hang too low and prematurely putting Plan C into effect. He decided I had a "need to know" that Dave was most likely going to make it home. So Matt kicked Plan C to the curb and I called Debbie to initiate Plan B. Even though all systems were already go for Matt's covert operation. My sweet Matt. I felt bad leaving him home, all alone, while we went out to celebrate on such a big night. I tried and tried to talk him into going with us but of course he wouldn't.

He couldn't. Inside, he must have been totally stressing out and trying to shove me out the door without me noticing, so he could make like crazy and whip that party into shape. But outside, he was nonchalant, telling me he'd just as soon keep his shirt on than go to a "topless restaurant, silly Mum." Did I mention he's a wise guy? Anyway, he said he'd be perfectly fine chilling, Facebooking, and playing Spider-Man.

Little did I know, when they pulled in the driveway to pick us up in Debbie's convertible, that Bob and Debbie were in cahoots with my Redheads for Operation T-A-P-A-S and that, I repeat, *everybody* was fully clothed. All the while my Redheads packed friends into the family room like so many snakes in a can (not that my friends are snakes or anything; it's just an analogy), ready to pounce and surprise the hell out of me.

We had a fabulous time at the tapas restaurant. Or I guess I should say I had a fabulous time. Dave and Debbie were frantically texting throughout dinner. Bob was distracted by what he thought was chocolate-drizzled tomatoes (it was balsamic vinaigrette, but the tomato part he got right) on his toast (flatbread). Bob was also a little bit disappointed at the portions. He's really tall and I could tell he was really hungry. I didn't think it was a good time to go into homeschool-mum-mode and to try and educate him about how "the idea" of tapas is really more about the people you're with than the portions, which are meant to be shared, BTW. I was neither frantic nor distracted, nor disappointed, but was blissfully oblivious—but that could have been the Spanish Quarter Cabernet-Tempranillo. I was on Spanish time, totally fiesta-ing, gearing up for a food-induced, Tempranillo-tempered siesta. And they were all trying to rush me, in the kindest way possible. There was, however, the tiniest of record scratches on the evening when I tried to order some crème brûlée, and they all practically wrestled the server to the ground for the bill, saying we'd stop off at Kroger and grab some ice cream to eat out on my back deck. I mean, don't get me wrong. I scream. You scream. We all do. I get it. But nothing says happy freaking cancerversary like dessert by blowtorch. Still I went along with them. Really, what choice did I have? Bob had driven.

The thing is, once we got in the car he forgot about the ice cream. I just sat there in the backseat with a forlorn look on my face as Bob drove. Right by. Kroger. Which sort of shocked me, since I knew he was still hungry. I can't remember if I cried or not. They completely ignored my puppy dog eyes and dragged me, not kicking but still screaming for ice cream, all the way home, just like the little piggy I was acting like. I didn't have a clue.

When we walked in the front door, I caught a glimpse of a candle burning in the bathroom on our way to the back deck. Sans ice cream, I might add.

"Why in the world does Matt have a candle burning downstairs when he's home alone?" I started to ask Dave.

But before I could even take a breath to signify the opening quotation marks, Dave saw the thought bubble over my head, and quickly popped it, by practically chest bumping me into the family room. And yes, as far as we can tell, they did in fact surprise the hell out of me.

Wow. Just wow. All I can say is that I was super glad I'd gone to the restroom at the tapas restaurant before we came home, or the most awesome surprise party *ever* wouldn't have been the only mark on this historic occasion in my life. Luckily, I'd asked to go before we left the restaurant. Which, at the time, I could tell got on their frantic nerves. And I think the only reason they let me go at all was because Debbie had to go, too. In the end, I'm sure everyone was quite as relieved as I was that they let me go.

And the party? It was one of those "having your cake and eating it too" kinds of nights. My Redheads and I did surgery on that cake and cut the cancer piece right out of the middle. Then we gave a short but sweet speech, after which we posed for a more innocent looking picture. What happened next was one forked up piece of cake. It wasn't a pretty sight. But it felt good.

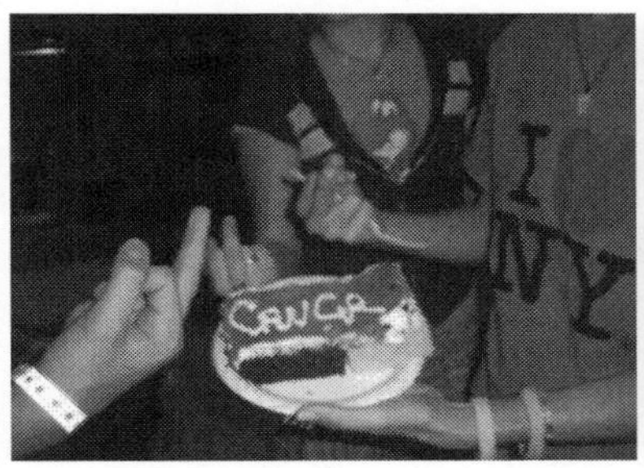

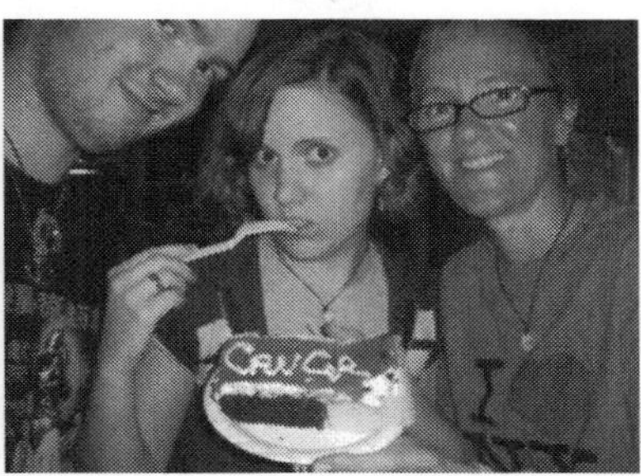

The next day, I dove into another year. It was time to whip the study into shape for our final year of homeschool. Also, that week, I had a chemo cocktail to down.

Once I'd downed Round 19, or T minus six, I only had *five chemo cocktails* to go! Which, as everybody knows, is a handful, but seemed so much more manageable to me than the twenty-four I had started out with, when I didn't even have enough numb fingers and soggy toes to keep count. I can't even begin to describe how ridiculously happy it made me to high-*five* everyone on my way out of the chemo cocktail lounge that day.

I continued to whip myself back into shape playing tennis. By this time I was playing singles matches on Tuesdays and doubles matches on Wednesdays. It was good to be back. And I was about eighty-five percent back, physically, though continuing to build stamina. I was still trying to deal with the way the port got in the way of my serve, and my soggy feet. But I was dealing. I had to buy a half-a-size-bigger shoe because my feet had developed claustrophobia. Even though I tricked them into roomier quarters, I still had to practically pry the shoes off after a match. I won't even tell you how matted my socks were to my feet or how I literally had to peel them off and then wring them out, because that's just TMI. Anyway, despite my complaining, my feet were happy feet to be playing tennis again, even if they were now ridiculously large. I reasoned that it made me that much harder to knock down.[45]

A couple of weeks after my mastectomy, I'd walked in my first Race for the Cure. So it was only appropriate that the 2009 Cincy race would follow on the heels of my cancerversary. Appropriately, some race volunteer gave me a hat that had one pink ribbon on it. I thought that was a pretty cool memento but I didn't wear it. I didn't feel like messing up my hair. Plus, honestly, I was over hats by then.

We gathered our team again, and a few of my new survivor friends walked with me. I'd written the names of friends who were fighting or had fought cancer on my race shirt: Sue, Linda, Stacy, Janet, Cathy, Kristi, Teri, Louise, Jo, Clusterfook, Deb, Judy and Chuck, Sue, Amy, Ron, Bill, Cheryl, Julie, Kay, Eileen, Cindy, and Vicki.

Sad how there seemed to be so many more people with cancer. Maybe I was just ultra aware. But I noticed that other people seemed to agree that pink was everywhere we turned, because breast cancer seemed to be turning up everywhere.

I wasn't in a post-surgical narcotic fog that year. Still, I found the solemnity of the event, which was magnified by the enormity of it all, to be ironically intoxicating.

One of my tennis girlfriends summed it up on her Facebook status: "If scientists had taken a satellite photo of downtown Cincinnati on Saturday, it would have shown a mysterious pink mist rising up. It was full of love and hope and friendship and courage, perseverance and faith, strength and gentleness. I was glad to be part of it."

I was hooked.

And if I wasn't high enough already, two weeks later I got to have another birthday. More still, as if I needed some icing on that cake, I got carded the night we went out for my forty-fourth birthday.

My dad always told me that two fours is a good roll in craps. Well, four-four was sure starting out like a good roll in life for me as well. My sister Jen had flown in from Charleston and she, Amanda, and I had a fabulous girls' night out for my birthday. We went to see a sneak preview of *Whip It* and rolled on the floor, laughing out loud, at how much Drew Barrymore reminded us of Jen, who left the movie smack-talking about joining the Charleston Roller Derby League when she returned home.

Since it was a sneak preview there was all kinds of hoopla and the theater was abuzz. They even threw free *Whip It* T-shirts out to the crowd, which I pretended was a birthday present to me. "T-shirts for everyone! On the house!" I was thinking as I pulled mine over the tank I was wearing, and then caught Amanda's mid-air and handed it to her.

After the movie and over much collaboration over T-A-P-A-S (in our *Whip It* shirts that we whipped on, not off) and a bottle of Spanish wine that I got carded for ordering, we all came up with roller derby names for ourselves. We decided we'd get them airbrushed on the backs of our T-shirts. Amanda would henceforth be Pandemic. (The name just rolled off her pet names, Amanda Panda Bear and Pandemonium). We tossed a coin over whether Jen should be heads: Jen and Tonic (my awesome idea) or tails: The Jenerator (Jen's idea). It was tails. I, of course, would henceforth be Chemosabe.

I couldn't wait to wear my new shirt to chemo.

Now if this book were an action film—which it's not (minus the Vespa incident)—this chapter would end a little like this: The new roller chick trio rolled out of the restaurant, posed, and fist-bumped the sky [cue theme song] and then off into the sunrise. But I'm pretty sure I wouldn't admit it.

---

[43] John 2

[44] "It's My Party and I'll Cry if I Want To"

[45] Weebles wobble but they don't fall down.

Rounds 20 through 22
Hey Joules

When I was hosting the Name My Port contest on my blog, all the while wearing down the etching on my Fear Not worry stone keychain that I carried with me *everywhere*, I should have seen the foreshadowing on the wall, in relation to the inherent tension between Port Rafa, my right pec, and me. By the time I was gearing up to down Round 20, the love–hate relationship between me and my port had been well established. Documented even. I'd come a long way from the days when I didn't want a port, to the day when my oncologist didn't give me a choice, to the day of the surgery when I joked about ports and pinot grigio, to the not-so-piece-of-cake days of recovery, to Port Rafa's first day on the job, to the nightmare of the Vespa incident, to the dog days of playing tennis with a port smack dab on my right pec.

I loved my port but only on chemo days, and only for purely selfish motives: to C.O.D. the chemo to the cancer. I'm OK if that makes me seem fickle. Port Rafa seemed OK with our working relationship. On tennis days, I hated it. I'm not even going to sugarcoat it. Most days were mostly a mixture of a smidgen of love and a streak of grrr, shaken and served with my twisted humor. Ambivalence is not one of my coping strategies. Living and loving like there's no tomorrow, and laughing my ass off, even in the face of cancer, are.

I know cancer isn't funny, but I believe it's OK to laugh when you have cancer. Even cancer patients need to laugh. Especially in the midst of serious cancer ass-kicking. Most cancer-ass-kicking breast surgeons, oncologists, survivors, and other superheroes I know agree with me that laughter doesn't cause cancer. Some say it even heals. (Bought that T-shirt too!) I'd really like to live to see the day we have the last laugh on cancer. I'd love to laugh all the way to a cure.[46] In the meantime, I've just got to laugh, despite the fact that cancer tried to kill me. I'm practicing my *mwahaha* for when we get there.

Right now it sounds a little scrawny I admit: a little like Simba, the lion-king-to-be, laughing in the face of danger. But to me, it's a whole lot more. I believe I'm in the midst of a divine comedy (in the classical sense) in that when the curtains close, there will be a happy ending. All questions will be answered. All loose ends tied up. Everything resolved. Everything will finally make sense. There will be no more tears.[47] Which is perfect, because like I said, I was born to laugh. Meanwhile, I'll do my Simba strut, cross the line, and trash-talk cancer till we find a cure.

Erma Bombeck penned, "There is a thin line that separates laughter and pain, comedy and tragedy, humor and hurt."

An extremely very fine line it seems to me. And I have issues with coloring within the lines as it is. Other than laughing so hard you cry, or at least till your stomach hurts, I can only think of one time that I was laughing one second and sobbing the next. It was odd, like our kids were, at the time (and by odd, I mean, of course, their ages: five, three, and one).

Well, one night after wrestling them all to bed, Dave wrestled me down to the ground and started tickling me. It ended up with me crying. I don't know why some people think other people like to be tickled because I don't know anybody over five who does. But that's not why I started crying.

I admit it, at first tickle I was caught off guard, and I did laugh. (It was before I got my much-hoped-for superpower of tickle resistance.) I laughed, not because it was funny or anything, but simply because I am freakishly ticklish. And I only laughed for a minute or so. A minute or so of tickling is thirty seconds too much for a contact sport, and gets old faster than a speeding bullet. Once I got to the point where I was gasping for air, my eyes, which had previously rolled back into my head from all the ROTFLOL-ing, managed to take a peek from flying their white flag of mercy. But do you think they saw mercy? In a word, no. Quite the contrary. What they saw was that everything I was doing was just egging Dave on. I think he must have misinterpreted those gasps for air for me blowing in his ear or something. The only thing left to do was tap into a latent layer of superpowers, the trifecta tickle defense: it's either squirm free, hyperventilate, or involuntarily rack the tickler.

I hate being tickled.

But I didn't employ any of the above. Instead—and I'm still not quite sure how this happened—somehow Dave must have flipped a cry switch I didn't even know I had. All of a sudden I was weeping. I don't know why. It was probably just exhaustion. Whatever. At least he stopped tickling me. And for the record, he felt *really* bad that it made me cry.

In tickling, I think it goes without saying that weeping is *not* the desired effect. Nobody means to tickle somebody's crying bone. Talk about raining on a parade. This is probably the most literal metaphorical example I can think of. But it serves as a good warning to ticklers everywhere: when laughter turns to tears, something has gone awry. A line has been crossed in a direction you didn't mean to go. So, why don'tcha tickle her fancy with champagne and dark chocolate instead? And anyway, tickling people's armpits is gross. So cut it out!

Luckily, this only happened to me once. However, I've experienced a reverse blurring of the lines quite a few times. The classic example is that scene in *Steel Magnolias* where M'Lynn is bawling her eyes out, screaming that she wants to hit somebody, and Clairee grabs Ouiser, pushes her forward, and says, "Here! Hit this! Go ahead, M'Lynn, slap her!" At which point, everybody (minus Ouiser), including the audience, dissolves into one of the best laughs ever to emanate from the silver screen. It's shocking. Disarming. Therapeutic. Addicting. As Truvy succinctly drawled, "Laughter through tears is my favorite emotion."

Which brings me back to the port-naming contest. I know it was silly. That was the point. Obviously, silliness is a precursor to laughter, and therefore, I think, a legitimate coping strategy. Yes, it was also a diversionary tactic. But it was more than merely a momentary distraction from everything that was happening. It was a means of escape. And by escape, I don't mean from reality. There was no escaping reality. Cancer was a big fat elephant in the middle of my living room. Que se-freaking-ra, sera. It was going to be what it was going to be. The question was, "What was I going to do with it?"

I totally could have thrown a fit, played the cancer card, and everybody would have cut me slack because they were all thinking, "poor Joules."

But I didn't feel like taking a chance on tapping into poor Joules and channeling that poor shrugging schmuck on the infamous orange Monopoly card for the rest of my life. It actually takes a lot more energy to maintain misery than I actually had after downing so many chemo cocktails. The fatigue hangover is the pits. And it's cumulative, so it's like that whole bowl of pits Erma Bombeck waxed on about in *If Life Is a Bowl of Cherries, What Am I Doing in the Pits*? If I had sat around wallowing in my misery thinking, "Poor me," that's exactly what would have happened. Misery loves company and I knew I could have had a giant pity party. But that sounded miserable. Dr. Lower's nurse, Brenda, pegged me pretty well when she playfully suggested I should name my port. I think she knew I'd play along and it must have flipped some kind of a switch in me. It even sounded kind of fun. I was so game. And the more the merrier, I got to thinking, so I invited my friends to play too. Thus, the contest was born.

I loved the name Port Rafa. But despite all my complaining, I'll be the first to admit that I couldn't have, wouldn't have, done chemo without it. Continuing the countdown at T minus five, we were on the same team if nothing else. Port Rafa had more than lived up to both meanings of its name, not to mention the theme song Amanda chose for it.

There couldn't have been a more perfect theme song for my port. When Amanda entered the contest, she practically delivered a doctoral thesis to me on why Hey Jude was so perfect. Due to space considerations in this less formal setting, here is her summary in her own words:

> So my mum had a contest in which she needed a name for her port, and I suggested Hey Jude. It's her favorite Beatles song and I always think of her when I hear it. Plus the lyrics were perfect: *take a sad song and make it better*. That's the kind of optimism my mum is into. Plus, you have to *let her into your heart* and *under your*

> *skin then you begin to make it better.* Awesome. Kind of like how the port has to be implanted under your skin into your heart path to inject the chemo which makes it better, better, better, *better....*

I was already a little better, being technically cancer free and all. But after I downed Round 20, I was even one step closer to better. The remaining four chemo cocktails were not exactly a cakewalk. Instead, they felt more like an awkward waltz, to rap music. I knew it might not look pretty, since I can't dance (wink, wink). But it felt so good to be so close to being done, to being better if you will, that I did a happy dance of sorts on my blog:

> I have only FOUR chemo cocktails left! Yay for the number FOUR! It's not a FOURgone conclusion, of course. Because in the FOURfront of my heart and mind, it is all, God willing, that I continue to move FOURward in this health and healing that he has mercifully and graciously FOURordained FOUR me; so without further ado, beFOUR I FOURget, I would like to thank him FOUR one more chemo cocktail in my rear-view mirror and this pleasant FOURshadowing of only FOUR more left. What a good gift that was for my FOURty-FOURth birthday! Makes my FOURhead unfurrow its brows as my smile tries to meet them. I won't go on about this FOURever, but I just thought I'd FOURwarn y'all, that in a wee bit more than a FOURtnight I will be teeing up FOUR the T minus FOURth and swinging like a mad woman. And I think you are supposed to yell "FOUR" when you do that. So FOUR! This post was brought to you by the number FOUR, obviously, but also by my new MacBook Pro that I got FOUR my birthday (along with its baby brother, my new iPhone) from my FOURmost supporter, Dave, who is usually not in the FOURfront, but behind the lines working overtimes to save up the dimes to support my writing and rhymes. How's that FOUR gangsta? Anyway, I just want to say thanks to the number FOUR, the peeps at Apple, Dave, and of course, FOUR viewers, like y'all!

Round 20 marked another three months on Herceptin so it was time for another MUGA scan. My heart was "all good," which made me feel even *better*. On top of me being radioactive and all.

I was barely done being radioactive, which this time came with a side of strep and bronchitis, when it was time to take Matt out for our famous night-before-a-birthday date. He was sixteen going on seventeen. After giving me a hard time about getting sick on his birthday and taking the spotlight off him, he brought me his own stash of Vicks VapoRub, because he was worried about me being all stuffy on our date. I was obviously not going to give or take a rain check. He was craving fried macaroni and cheese so we headed to Friday's.

As soon as the server took our order, I flipped over my placemat and traced our hands, wrote the date, and we had the same Q&A session that we'd had every night before a birthday every year since Amanda's night-before-her-fourth birthday. Thirteen years of the most precious data I've ever had the pleasure to collect. Wow. I highly recommend interviewing one's children regularly. When I asked him the high–low of the year, he shocked and awed me, humbled me, by saying *cancer* for both.

"It's definitely *the* con," he explained, "but in a way, it's also been a pro, because even though it sucked, we needed it. I don't really remember what it was like before the cancer but I think it brought us all closer together. And it helped me realize it's so much easier to just trust God rather than take things into your own hands. Because cancer isn't something you can take in your hands, and you just have to trust God."

Wow. Just wow. Even if I wasn't already practically laryngitic, I was speechless then. As far as mommy moments go, there are no words. Just Mary's example of treasuring up things in her heart.[48]

I can only imagine what my sweet kids went through having to help care for such a very sick mum, who was supposed to be the one taking care of them. This was not in my mum's manual, nor my intended homeschool curriculum.

Cancer was definitely a game-changer, or maybe I'd say more of a fine-tuner. Cancer wasn't the center of our lives, but it did center our lives. Cancer was that elephant in the middle of the room that you really can't ignore. So you just feed it peanuts and get on with life as much as you can, with an elephant following you around wherever you go, begging for more peanuts.

The cool thing about my Redheads is that they somehow figured out how to ride the elephant. At least that's the way it seemed to me, and that made me laugh, and it gave me courage. It seemed to make things a little better, even in the middle of cancer.

After the fried macaroni and cheese, Matt wanted to see *Surrogates* and I was glad to be the one to take him. He likes action flicks, and I was OK with the idea of chilling at the movies. The craziest, coolest thing happened during the movie though, which made it feel like I was getting a present on Matt's birthday. Out of the blue I got an email asking me to write an article for breast cancer awareness month for ChristianityToday.com.

B-E-T-T-E-R

But wait, there was more: T minus 4, T minus 3, Rounds 21 and 22. Better, better.

And last but not least, there was the unexpected delight of chemo cocktail communion with a survivor sister I'd met on my birthday, when she was doing her first Tax-ALL/Herceptin cocktail. There's this crazy instant connection survivors have. Chemo cocktails are thicker than water, so I totally get it if others get a little jealous. But Shelly and I were like, if you'll excuse the expression, two peas in a pod. You know I have a general disgust for peas and so it most likely catches you off guard that I'd stoop to use the reference. I totally get what you're saying, but in this *sole* instance, it just works. Especially when you have communion over a half-dozen chemo cocktails. Chemo is definitely thicker than water.

Better. Nah nah nah nah. Hey Joules. Yeah! Waaahhh!

---

[46] Proverbs 17:22

[47] Revelation 21:4

[48] Luke 2:19

Round 23
This Is Country Music

The doctor wasn't supposed to say the word *cancer*. But dammit, she did.

And I know you're not supposed to say *dammit* in a book where you just said Jesus is the answer for your cancer, either. But *dammit*.

Damn cancer.

That's right. I just said *damn cancer*. And I mean it.

(What I don't mean to do, however, is offend anybody. So I am really sorry about that if I did. It's just that I don't do pretense very well and *dammit* is pretty much how I feel about cancer. I actually think Jesus feels the same way, if you want to know the truth, because in the end that's exactly what he's going to do with it. Jesus is going to damn cancer and send it straight to hell. Which is one reason I don't mind saying he rocks, in a chapter with a country music song title, even if you're not supposed to say so. So be it. Which is as much to say, amen.)

And, ahem, as I was saying, *damn cancer*.

I know the doctor saying the word *cancer* is last thing you wanted me to say this close to the end of the book, and if you only knew how much I hated having to write it, you'd probably buy me a beer to cry in. I know what you're thinking, too. "But you weren't even done with chemo yet. That's not even fair." Exactly. I wasn't. It wasn't.

But it's not *exactly* what you're thinking. Part of me wished it were, in a way. But when I was sitting in the doctor's office that day, surrounded by my mum and aunties and a few close friends, it wasn't *my* doctor who said the *C* word.

It was *my mum's*.

Dammit. Dammit.

When I downed T minus three I could count my remaining chemo cocktails on two fingers, which everybody knows is the universal sign for peace. Everybody that is, except cancer. But I guess it shouldn't surprise any of us that cancer doesn't play by the rules.

We all know the statistics: one in eight women will be diagnosed with cancer of the breast during their lifetime.[49]

If I was one of the one in eight, then I felt like I oughta, at the very least, get to call dibs that my daughter, my sister, and my mum get to be counted part of the "other seven."

Damn cancer.

Now my mum had been dealing with some health issues, the main ones (we thought) being Bell's palsy and some abscessed teeth. T minus three, for me, happened in the middle of a mass of doctor's appointments for her. She didn't even tell me about the two mammograms she had had that came back warranting a biopsy, until practically the day before the biopsy. Which was the day after my T minus three. She'd been trying to spare me unnecessary stress, and so had up till then neglected telling me about the mammograms.

Speaking of mammograms, you'd think that as soon as I got diagnosed, everybody and their sister would have stood in line to get one. Well, everybody did but my mother. She doesn't have health insurance and therefore doesn't really do doctors much.

Thank God for Little Red Door Cancer Agency, is all I can say.[50]

My mum happened to be watching TV when they aired a news segment about offering free mammograms, which she happened to catch, which happened to move her to making an appointment. Thank God.

The fact that all this happened the very same week that the new (though quickly outdated) guidelines for mammograms came out was as infuriating as it was ironic.[51]

I'd just like to point out that I would not be typing these words if I had waited until I turned fifty to have my first mammogram. To put it bluntly, I'd be dead if I hadn't had the mammogram, which saw the red flag flying.

T minus three went down on a Monday. Wednesday, my mum had the biopsy. Friday I drove to Indy, and there we were, sitting in her doctor's office waiting for the word.

The doctor was not supposed to say the *C* word.

Even my genetic test results echoed "No freaking way!"

Damn cancer.

If only it had the tact, or at the very least, mercy, to wait until I was done downing chemo cocktails. It would have been nice to feel stronger, to be stronger for my mum in the midst of her own cancer. But like I said, cancer isn't fair.

Luckily, we'd caught it early.

"Early diagnosis, excellent prognosis!" I could practically hear Dr. Lower cheering all the way from Cincinnati.

It was really the best news we could hope for. My mum's doctor said it was non-invasive ductile carcinoma, and staged it at 0. It was a cluster of cancer cells, in a duct, that we were going to be able to stop in their tracks before the cancer could spread further.

The game plan we settled on was a lumpectomy, followed up with thirty-three rounds of radiation.

Not many mums go that far in sympathizing with their daughters. But my mum did.

A couple of weeks later I continued my own chemo cocktail countdown, at T minus two, tossing back Round 23.

OMG, I only had one round left! Can I even tell you how happy it made me to finally be able to say that? They may say that one is the loneliest number, but not me, myself, and I. Especially when it comes to chemo cocktails.

I don't know if it was some kind of chain reaction after downing T minus two, or if it was in honor of the peace sign I'd flashed that day, but two incredible, unbelievable things happened to me after that.

First, I had the honor of paying forward the Tiffany Award I'd received the previous year, to the 2009 recipient, Mary Jo Cropper. A humbling experience to say the least, considering it was *the* Mary Jo of what is now called the Mary Jo Cropper Family Center for Breast Care at Bethesda North Hospital in Cincinnati, where I'd had my own mammogram.

So in a way, she'd saved my life.

How lucky was I to be able to thank her?

A few days later—I can't even believe I get to say this—but both my singles and doubles teams made it to the Greater Cincinnati Tennis Association play-offs!

My singles team came in second both for the season and in the play-offs. I got pummeled in the play-offs by my friend Jamie. The thing about Jamie is that she is one of the sweetest people in the world, and you'd never guess that she'd get into beating cancer patients in tennis like she does. But then again, she'd be the first one to buy you a beer afterward, lift one with you, and toast to your health. So it's kind of hard to stay mad at her for very long.

Despite that thumping, I ended the season with an 8-3 record.

My doubles team *won the play-offs!* We came in first in our division, but were the definite underdogs going into the play-offs. There were seventeen teams in all. The top three from each division made it to play-offs, and then a fourth team with the next highest points got a wild card entry. Even the wild card team had more points than my team did. I'm pretty sure the team we played in the first round match not-so-secretly breathed a sigh of relief when they drew us, since they'd beaten us 8-1 during the season. I think the other finalist team also breathed a sigh of relief when they got to play us instead of the top-seeded team for the championship, since they had also beaten us during the season, 6-3.

I think we surprised everyone else as much as we surprised ourselves. In the end, I have to say this about an amazing aspect of women's tennis: practically everybody was cheering for me and my team. I mean, who can't get on board and cheer an underdog like that? What a comeback season!

And what an exclamation point on my recovery! I totally channeled Rafa and took a bite out of the trophy.

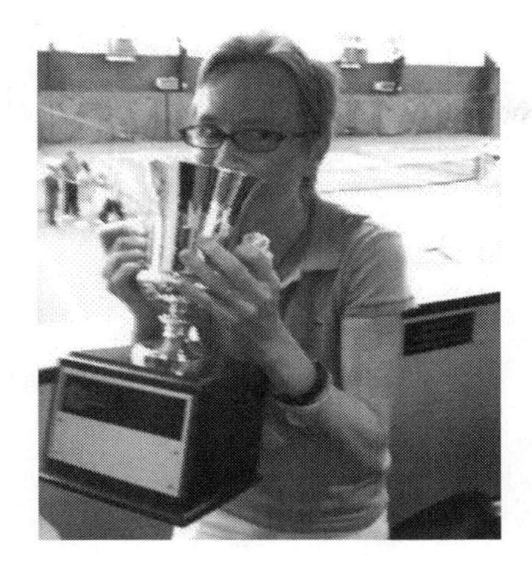

We totally rocked! But I suppose you're not supposed to say that in a chapter about country music. Oh. What the hell. It's how I roll.

---

[49] http://www.breastcancer.org/symptoms/understand_bc/statistics.jsp

[50] http://www.littlereddoor.org/

[51] http://www.mayoclinic.com/health/mammogram-guidelines/AN02052

Round 24
Cancer Was a Bitch

It was almost Christmas, and thank God I got to be there. (By *there*, I wasn't exactly meaning the chemo cocktail lounge where I was downing MY LAST ROUND, if you know what I mean.) When you're still recovering from hearing the *C* word, and on top of that a mastectomy, and then your eyes go *boi-oi-oing* because you're standing there one against two dozen chemo cocktails, it's almost enough to make you crack before you even begin. And when you're sitting there, shaking in your boots like that, twenty-four might as well have a line over it, with an ellipsis in its wake. It feels that......................far....................................away.

But here it was, almost Christmas again. And this year, I felt like I was at the top of Santa's nice list because I was getting no more chemo. For good. And how.

Bartender, I'd had enough.

It had sure been one helluva year. Yeah, thank God I was there.

Since it was beginning to look a lot like Christmas, of course I wore my Santa Claus hat and brought some elves with me to the chemo cocktail lounge to help me count down and celebrate. They caroled the chemo lounge.

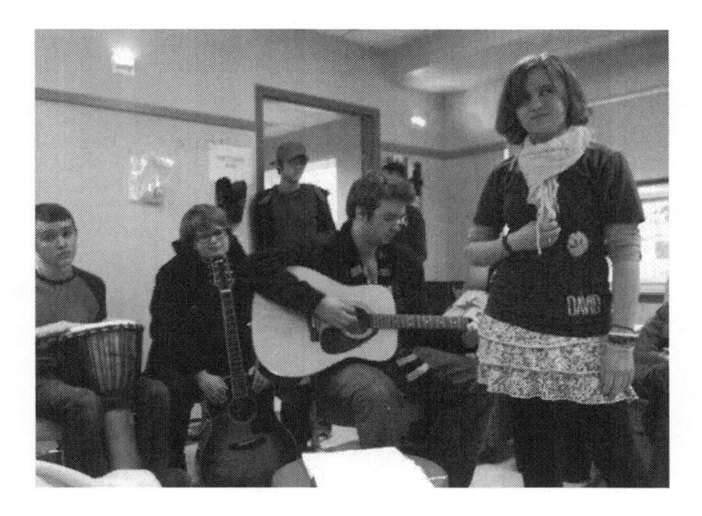

My favorite carol was one my Redheads had written for me, to celebrate my last chemo cocktail.

The Chemo Cocktail Song
(or Cancer Is a Bitch)

By The Kicked-In Fence[52]
Lyrics by Amanda, Matt, and Mikeyy Evans
Music by Matt Evans

It's Christmas again
And thank God you're here
Christmas again
It's been one helluva year
Yeah, thank God you're here
And didya bring out your hair
Your head's awfully nice
Even when it's bare

Refrain
Don't wanna go to chemo
I don't wanna go

Chorus
Well, cancer's a bitch
But you're stronger than it is
Yeah, cancer's a bitch

So let's kick it in the ditch
You can fall asleep
In your chemo chair
I'll buy you a wig
Or maybe draw on some hair

Take off your gloves
You'll box here no more
The only drinks left
Will leave you out on the floor

Refrain
Chorus
Well cancer's a bitch
But you're stronger than it is
Yeah, cancer's a bitch
Let's kick it in the ditch
Kickin' it in the ditch
Yeah, you've kicked it in the ditch

Well cancer's a bitch
It wasn't a cinch
Repeat xxx

Well, some have gone before
And their eyelids met peace
But I'll find you in dreams
'Cause in his arms you will sleep.

That's right, my sweet, petite, redheaded hippie child wrote me a theme song called "Cancer Is a Bitch." Yeah, we're probably not your average homeschool family.

There weren't many dry eyes in the room. When Amanda got to the chorus for the first time, it was one of those *Steel Magnolias* moments.

"Did she just say *bitch*? Yeah, I think that's what she just said. Oops, she said it again. Wow, I don't think I've ever heard that word sound so . . . beautiful. But yeah, she's right. Cancer *is* a bitch." And then, the applause and the amens broke out.

Laughter through tears—it's a beautiful thing, especially in the middle of chemo.

I was sitting next to my chemo sister, Shelly, who was downing her last Taxol, while I downed my last Herceptin.

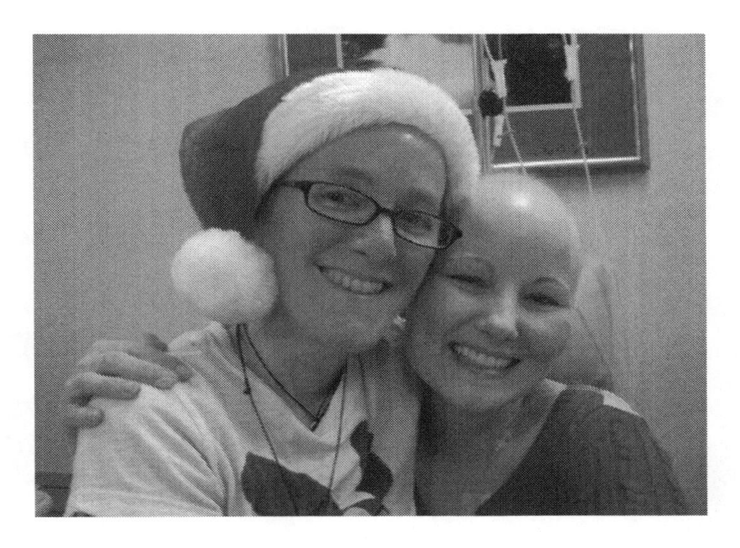

She'd get to down her last chemo cocktail in September. There was a part of me that had a hard time celebrating, like I was bragging that I was done or something. I know that was silly, and I know Shelly was celebrating with me as much as I was with her, through the laughter and tears of her own fight. She and her daughters, Savannah and Audrey, had even made Christmas cookies for my end-of-chemo party at the chemo cocktail lounge. Never have fork marks in a peanut butter cookie been so sweet. And you should have tasted the Hershey's Kiss in each one.

In response to the song, I even brought my hair. It looked like someone had shaken salt and pepper on my head. I guess you could call it well seasoned if you feel like being poetic like I do sometimes. Either way, I was done with chemo. Not in the well-done sense, although I hope the chemo did a good job in the well-done sense.

Anyway, nobody wants to go to chemo. People complain about having to vote between the lesser of two evils during every election. But elephants and donkeys got nuthin' on cancer and chemo as far as I'm concerned. And that is about as political as I get. I didn't want to go to chemo, but it was *the* legit lesser evil. Like my sister said when she came to chemo with me one time, "It's hard to get over the fact that they are dripping poison in your IV. It's hard to get over the fact that *that's* what it takes to kick cancer's ass."

So I downed the last chemo cocktail.

Then, we packed Yukon and headed for a balmy Christmas at the beach. Besides no more chemo, all I really wanted for Christmas was to take a little holiday with my little family, somewhere where I could walk barefoot in the sand.

Santa delivered.

Here was my Happy New Year's Day post(card) from the road:

> The wisest man in the world once wrote about there being a time for everything that happens down here, under heaven…[53]
>
> *There's a time to be born—*
> Today a new year is born. 2010, the year of my Lord, whose birth I just celebrated last week.
>
> *And a time to die—*
> 2009 was not my time although between cancer and the Vespa incident I know I kept everyone worried, and even I wondered a couple of times. 2009 was the time for my Gramcracker and I really miss her but I am so happy that she got to hang out with Jesus on his birthday.
>
> *A time to plant—*
> Amanda turned eighteen, entering into adulthood and her sophomore year as a journalism major at University of Cincinnati. We "planted" her in a cute little apartment on campus to eliminate the commute from her life and to open the door for her on college life. Also, we had already been blooming at the Cincy Vineyard, but we officially "planted" ourselves there by becoming members.

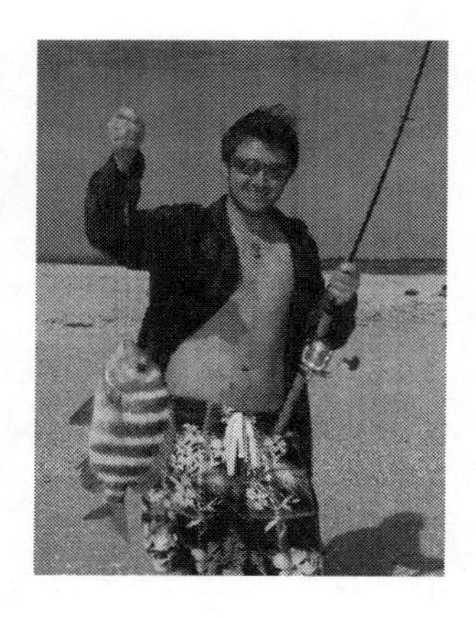

And a time to reap—
In 2009, Dave's company, 3dB Labs, turned five years old. Just like the Life Is Good motto, God has provided Dave the opportunity to be able to "do what you like and like what you do" in his "hunting and gathering" part of providing for our family. And this year, for the first time, he did actually get to reap a bit of the fruit of his labor, from whose hands we know all blessings flow, and to whom we are eternally grateful.

A time to kill—
2009 was a year of killing cancer cells in me. Our calendar has literally revolved around my chemo cocktail schedule. Twenty-four rounds over the past year and a half. I have felt like such a hobbit through it all. I had no idea I had it in me to do this adventure of slaying dragons and such, but I have had the best company a hobbit could hope for. And now that we have gone there and back again being back again feels like a whole new adventure.

And a time to heal—
I am looking forward to 2010, to laying down weapons and to the turning over aloe leaves and a whole new set of leaves on a brand new calendar.

A time to break down—
Four rounds of The Red Devil and Cytoxan, a derivative of mustard gas. Four rounds of taxing Tax-ALL. Nineteen rounds of Herceptin.

And a time to build up—
A generous gift from The Tiffany Foundation of a membership to my tennis club to help me regain my fitness as I recover my health. They are a delightful group of women to play tennis with. They helped me get my game back and we won play-offs to boot!

A time to cry—
There have been sad tears :"(
But. there have been happy ones, too :")
And honestly, more of those sad ones have been from Amanda cutting my freaking apron strings than from the cancer. I have tasted my own salty tears through it all but I think God has been my ever present help in time of need to wipe them away and to leave me with an aftertaste of that peace that passes understanding. The happy ones have mainly been the overflow

of treasuring all things Redheads in my heart. I have loved every stage of my kids' growth, but I have to admit that I LOVE this present stage of their becoming and blooming. They are good and godly peeps, and the sweet hearts of my heart.

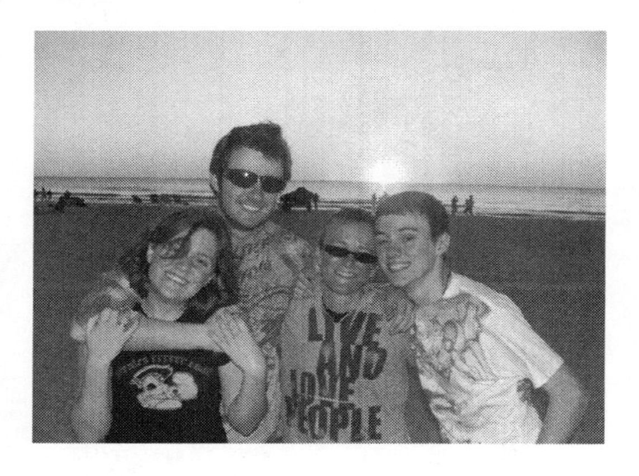

And a time to laugh—
The Evanshire is a hobbit hole full of wise guys. Sometimes it feels like we are in a sitcom. But the thing is, we do love to laugh. And we do laugh a lot.

A time to have sorrow—
I wouldn't necessarily have chosen the cup of suffering I have been sipping from this past year and a half. But I do trust God, the one through whose hands I believe the cup was given to me, for his glory, and my good. I know there are some who would disagree with me on that statement, and I'm not trying to pick a theological debate here. It's just that I find more comfort in believing he handed me the cup than that the devil handed it to me behind his back or against his will. I also believe that joy comes in the morning and that my time of mourning will be turned into . . .

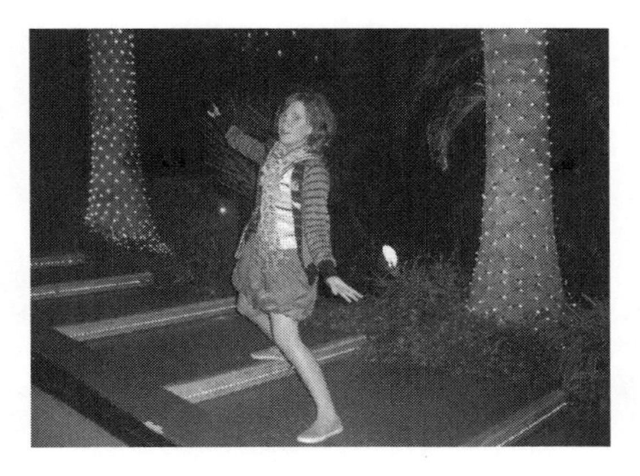

A time to dance—
We got the *Let's Dance* game for the Wii for Christmas, so we should be set.

A time to throw stones—
I haven't really been able to throw at all with Port Rafa sitting on my right pec muscle. It has really cramped my range of motion, which in turn put a kink my tennis serve. I have totally had to improvise a new serve to be able to compete. It doesn't have much pace on it, but I can consistently get it in the box. Still, I'm looking forward to having Port Rafa removed on Wednesday, which also happens to be Epiphany. Bon freaking voyage! Then, I will THROW a non-chemo cocktail party on Friday, January 8, to really celebrate the end, God willing, of my cancer chapter!

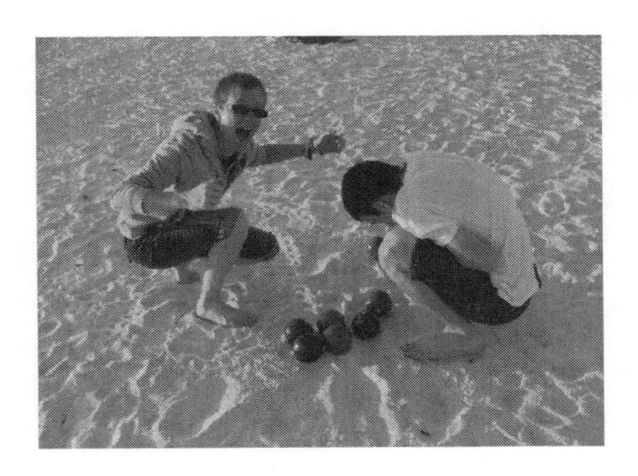

And a time to gather stones—
One of the coolest things that my boys did for me while I was sick was to gather stones and make a path for me down to the tennis courts behind the Evanshire. I'm looking forward to wearing down that path with Mikeyy when spring springs. We'll see if this is the year he leaves me in his tennis wake.

A time to kiss—
Our twenty-second anniversary and another New Year's Eve. We celebrated both while on holiday, which was the light at the end of the chemo tunnel for us all. Also, there are Hershey's Kisses. And I just secretly wonder if we all gathered Hershey's Kisses (especially the kind with peanut butter inside) instead of stones, and if we didn't throw them, but gave them to one another....
Well, that would be sweet.

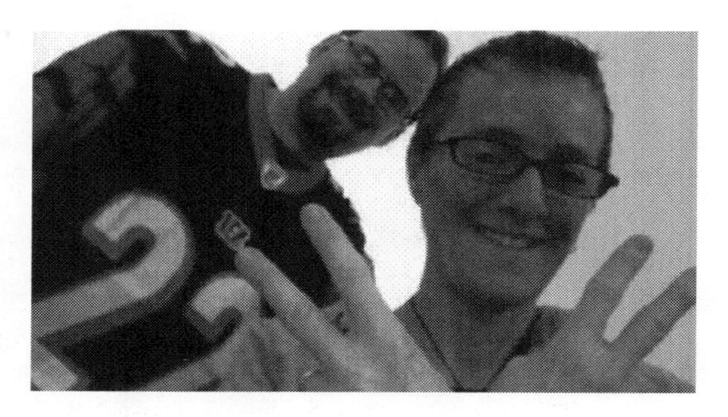

And a time to turn from kissing—
Morning breath is a good example of this refraining refrain. And here is where a Hershey's Kiss could really come in handy in the clutch.

A time to try to find—
This past week we found Marco (Island) before he could say Polo. In other words, we took a much-needed family holiday away from the cancer and the chemo of this past year and a half of our life.

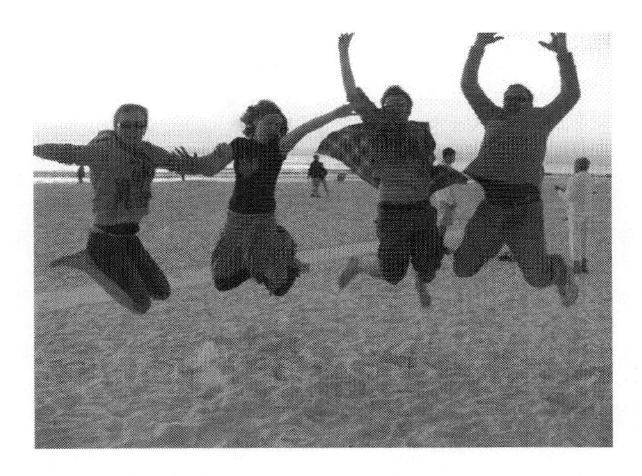

And a time to lose—
We have lost a lot over the past year and a half. A pound (give or take) of my flesh, Dave's gall bladder, my Gramcracker, my friend Linda, my hair and taste buds during chemo and even some of the feeling in my feet and fingertips, my old computer, the clutch on my Mini, three cameras, and I definitely lost face in Rome, not to mention my opportunity to put my hand in the Mouth of Truth, when I crashed into a wall. Coincidentally, the wall was made of stones someone had gathered; either that, or the Vespa got confused and threw me. Anyway, we didn't lose time in going on holiday the very next day after my very last chemo.

A time to keep—
Time. Is Precious. Can't really keep it (don't really have rhythm, either) but being in the moment and making memories are my kind of keepsakes.

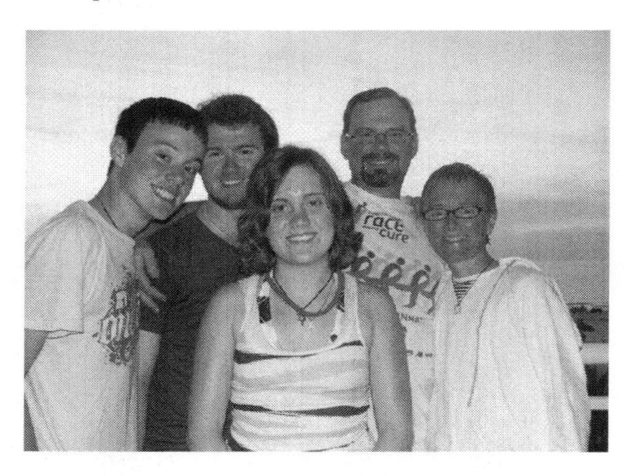

And a time to throw away—
When Port Rafa sails away on Wednesday, I won't need the instruction manual anymore. I am giving it back to the surgeon. No, I didn't read it. It was just TMI for me but I think Dave read it.

A time to tear apart—
God willing, Wednesday will be the last surgery I need for a very long time.

And a time to sew together—
And I'm looking forward to being sewn back together, sans port, then piecing back together my serve. Maybe even throwing a few stones, and by throwing, I mean skipping stones that I have gathered. But never when there is a glass house in the background.

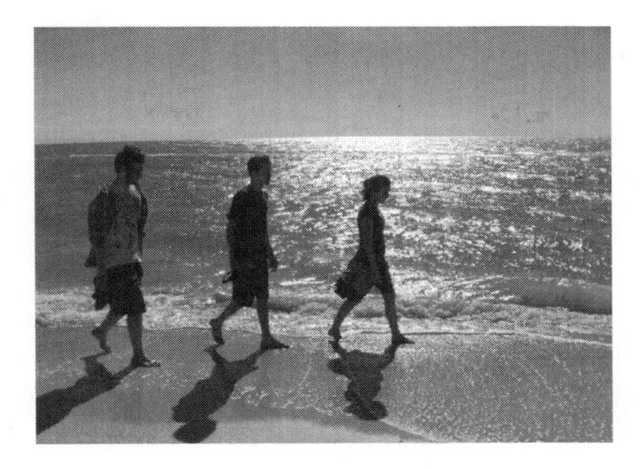

A time to be quiet—
One time that immediately pops into my mind was the surprise party my kids threw me for my one-year anniversary of being cancer free. I still don't know how they pulled that off.

And a time to speak—
Obviously I pulled this one off with this lengthy post(card) from the other side of breast cancer and chemo. But the main thing I hope that it says loud and clear is thank You, God. And may the rest of my life say the same thing. Also, I'd like to say thank you, again, to everyone for all the prayers and acts of kindness that have helped carry me there and back again. Truly I've gotten by "with a little help from my friends."

A time to love—
The rest of my time.

And a time to hate—
Been there, done that. Hated it.

A time for war—
Bought the T-shirt. Cancer sucks.

And, a time for peace.
Selah.

And with that, it was finally five o'clock in my cancer battle, not to mention this book. Time to hang up my pink boxing gloves. Time to make our glasses overflow. (Of course, I had mine shaken not stirred.) Time to lift our glasses and thank God we're still here. Time to clink those glasses together and say, "Cheers!"

---

[52] http://www.myspace.com/thekickedinfence

[53] King Solomon, Ecclesiastes 3

Part III – Hangover

P.S.

Beautiful Things

So I just want to thank you for hanging in there with me till the "happily ever after" part of my book. I know I promised you a comedy about my tragedy and well, here we are—and here I am—still typing! But you already knew that since I gave it away back when I broke down (because I was worrying about you, gentle reader, worrying about me) and gave you the spoiler alert in the "Backwards" chapter. I hope that didn't ruin the ending for you because the last thing I feel about being at the end of my very first book is anticlimactic.

I also hope you laughed, being that this is a comedy, or it's too bad for me since I quit my day job.

Now I know this is the part where I'm *supposed* to leave you hanging on the proverbial cliff, so to speak, so you'll wonder what happens next—and—once you close the book you'll feel compelled to rush out and buy my next one . . . *but* . . . well, for one thing that just seems cruel to leave people dangling like that. The other thing is…I don't know what happens next.

I mean, I know beautiful things have happened, are happening, and will happen.

Port Rafa did indeed sail away on January 6, 2010, and my ecstatic right pec said bon freaking voyage! For some reason Dave wanted to keep my port—since we paid so much for it and all. I thought it was a pretty sick idea, but I ended up taking in a nice bottle of port and traded Dr. Runk for it, for Dave. I thought it was the least I could do. Though, I personally think Dr. Runk got the better end of the deal. But then again, she probably deserved a drink after having to dig Port Rafa out from under such well-developed tennis pectoral muscles. It was the least I could do.

After Port Rafa bon voyaged, which was, for me, the emphatic closure on my chemo cocktail tab, it was, of course, a time for a party. So a couple of days later I threw a Not a Chemo Cocktail Party to end all chemo cocktail parties bash. This time, I did buy the flowers and the wine. And I got to thank all my friends proper. Well, as much as you can. There's no way, really, that I can think to pay them all back, except by paying it forward. Which is how I intend to spend myself all the rest of my days. It's the least I can do.

A month after the port was removed, I had my post-chemo-and-hopefully-cancer scans, after which, I penned the following on my blog:

> My Redheads shook their heads and gave me that "silly mum" look when I told them that as soon as I finished my last scan yesterday, I threw the nuclear medicine doors wide open and ran down the long hallway to the waiting room where Dave was doing Sudoku and waiting for me.
>
> Once the doors closed behind me and it was just me in that long, hollow corridor, I couldn't help but throw up my arms, say "YES!" from the very depths of my soul, and then sprint out of there.
>
> From the waiting room we decided that waiting was for the birds, rolled the dice, passed Go, and went to collect the X-rays and reports.
>
> I will cut to the chase and say that while we haven't talked to my oncologist yet and gotten her professional opinion and official word, the reports clearly say that from head to toe and inside-out, there is no evidence of metastatic disease in me! God has truly had mercy on me. By his wounds I am healed. Amen.

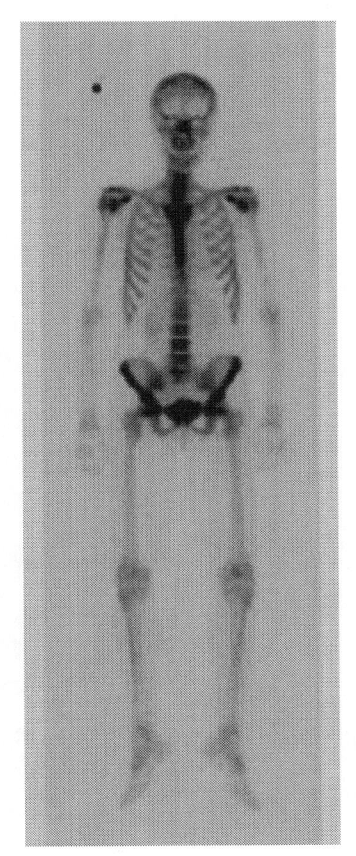

Dem bones be me
Dem bones be cancer free!
Dem bones be dancing
Like the Hand of God be upon me,
Doing a jig to Ezekiel's tune
That He sang in the Valley of the Dry Bones.[54]
Dem bones dance for Him.

At that point I could have said "The End" but to me it really felt more like flipping back to the beginning and starting over, a whole new "Once Upon a Time..."

So obviously "The End" doesn't really work in this particular case, and thus this tale ends up without a tail. It seems fitting that Eeyore should have the last word in this chemo cocktail of mine: "It's not much of a tail, but I'm sort of attached to it."

[54] Ezekiel 37:1-10

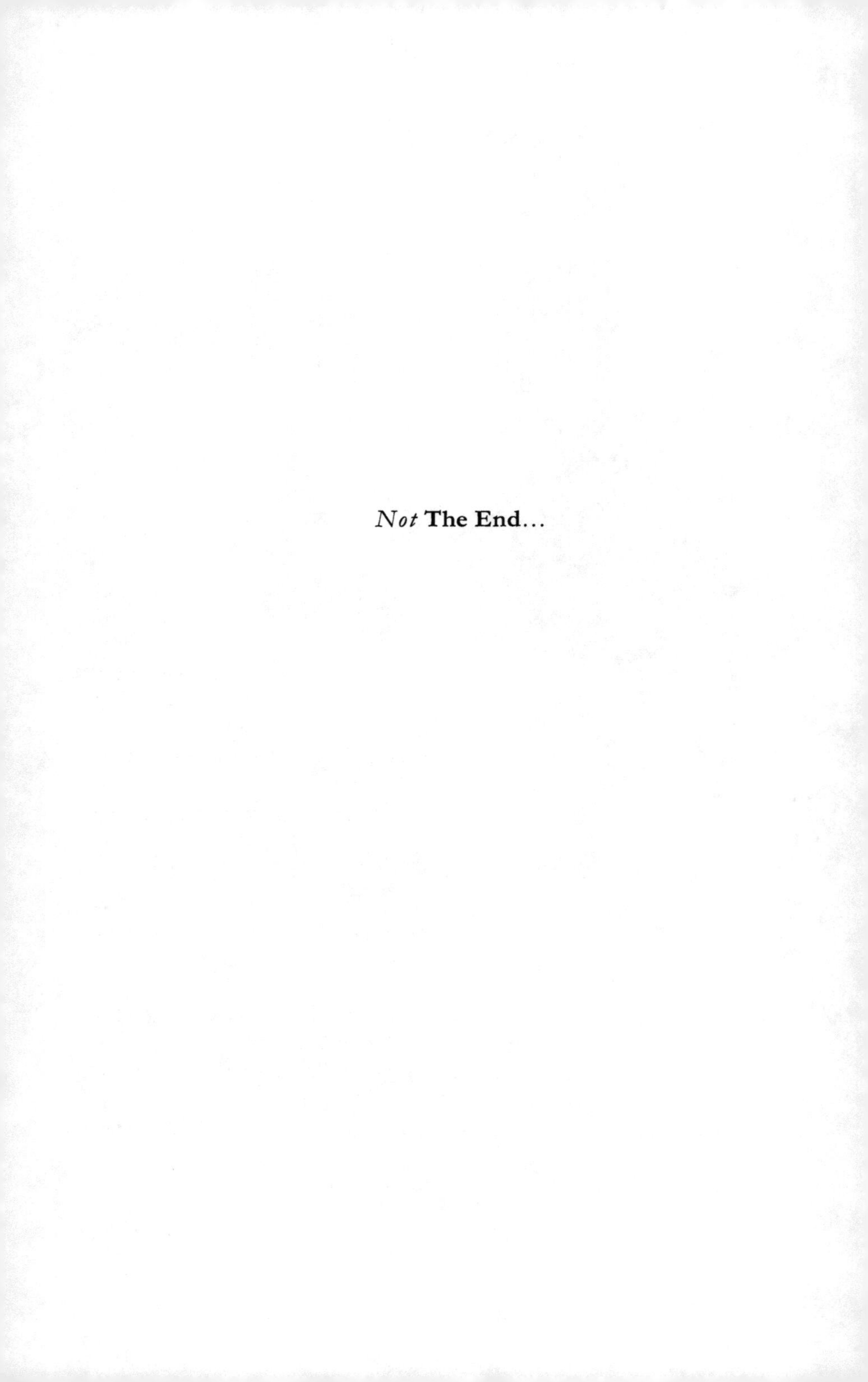

Not **The End…**

XOXO

Thank you God for the gift of second chances at life, and for the satisfaction of sensing your pleasure when I write.

Thank you Dave, Amanda, Matt, and Mikeyy for going there and back again with me. And thank you for reading it over and over and helping me edit the manuscript. Thank you Mikeyy for being my graphic design guru for the book and my soundmix man for the audio book. Thanks Redheads for the "Cancer Is a Bitch" song.

Thank you Dr. Allen, Dr. Stahl, Rita, Sharon, Dr. Runk, Dr. Lower, Brenda (and all the crew at the Taft office of Oncology Hematology Care) for being the best cancer ass-kicking team a girl could ask for.

Thank you Jen, my baby sister and best friend, for flying all the way to Cincinnati when I needed you most, and for always being there for me in Charleston, by the beach, to boot!

Thank you Debbie and Celina for organizing pretty much everything behind the scenes to take care of me and my family and for being the kinds of friends who stick close when your sister lives in Charleston.

Thank you all my friends for being the most amazing support system in the history of the world. Never has "I Get By With a Little Help from My Friends" ever been so true.

Thank you to everyone who brought meals to the Evanshire during chemo weeks.

Thank you Alton, Pete, and the Vineyard Student Union for loving on my Redheads.

Thank you Dave's Iron Men for supporting Dave through everything and Dan Henry for bringing me communion before my mastectomy.

Thank you Dave Workman and Joe Boyd, my pastors at Vineyard Cincinnati, whose faithful teaching helped me keep my hope and perspective afloat.

Thank you to the small group that meets at the Evanshire for your friendship and for praying with us through my cancer battle.

Thank you prayer team of Vineyard Cincinnati for praying over me for healing every week throughout my cancer battle.

Thank you Lisa Demaree for praying for the bald chick at church every week.

Thank you Learning Tree Mums for praying over me before chemo.

Thank you Julie Sweeney for your friendship and for being my sidekick/support in Brit Lit class.

Thank you Cathy for lending me your hats when I was bald.

Thank you Nancy and Toots for being my phone-a-friend oncology nurses.

Thank you Tiffany Foundation and Five Seasons and Team Green for helping me regain my fitness and get back out on the tennis courts.

Thank you Kristi. You are a postcard from hope.

Thank you Jamie for our tennis match and for taking me under your wings.

Thank you Karen Wellington Foundation for all the encouragement to not just survive but thrive and for sending Dave and I to Cancun after my cancer battle that had hijacked our twentieth-anniversary Caribbean holiday.

Thank you Juliet for being my angel in Rome.

Thank you Shelly for being such a ray of sunshine when you walked into the chemo cocktail lounge and my life, chemo sister.

Thank you Becky Johnson for letting me see how writing a book is done and then encouraging me to do it.

Thank you Anne Lamott for your "Instructions on Writing and Life." Who knew that when I read about you looking for a "funny book about cancer" I would end up writing my own "illuminate the experience and make me laugh." I wrote it just like you taught, *Bird by Bird.*

Thank you Gail Konop Baker and Geralyn Lucas for writing funny books about cancer that made me laugh when I needed it most. And cheers to both of you, and your health.

Thank you Mt. Hermon for an amazing writing conference which was my diving board into this book.

Thank you Lynn Vincent for your narrative nonfiction track at Mt. Hermon, for the gift of your time there, and for encouraging me.

Thank you Mike and Christy Williams of Book Bums for my writers group, the Word Bums of Book Bums, and for being the most amazing support system throughout the writing of this book. Thank you Christy for reading it as I wrote, and for cheering me on.

Thank you London for making me a cartoon. I always wanted to be a cartoon!

Thank you Sara Huron of Wide Margins (www.widemargins.com) for editing the manuscript. Oops, I so almost tattooted!

Thank you Julia Fikse for starting www.savethetatas.com, for your passion in the fight against cancer, but also for "putting some fun in the fight against cancer." Thank you for reading my first draft, for your feedback and encouragement, and most of all your friendship.

Thank you David Jay for The SCAR Project exhibit. Thank you for the honor and pleasure of working with you (and Sandie) to bring the exhibit, which premiered in New York City, to Cincinnati. Your artistic integrity and ingenuity has been a source of inspiration as I've portrayed my absolute reality of surviving cancer in the portrait of the lady in this memoir.

Thank you to my SCAR Project Cincinnati Exhibit committee: Vanessa Tiemeier, Litsa Spanos, Pam Irvin, Shelly Emrick, Banita Bailey. Such beautiful souls. One of the most meaningful things I've ever done.

Thank you Litsa Spanos. There really are no words to express my deep gratitude for helping me and Vanessa bring The SCAR Project to Cincinnati. You are the most generous soul I know. How lucky am I to have you in my life.

Thank you to all The SCAR Project girls who came to Cincinnati to the exhibit. I admire you for "Baring It All" for The SCAR Project, revealing the absolute reality of surviving cancer in order to help raise awareness. Your beauty, strength, courage, and grace inspires me. May it both save lives and be traction for a cure. Cheers to all of you, and to your health.

In memory of Sue, Linda, Yott's mum, Maria Meyer, Gramcracker, Tiffany, Karen Wellington, Mary Jo Cropper, Heather Ray, Kaye, Sue, Amy, Andy, and Jolene

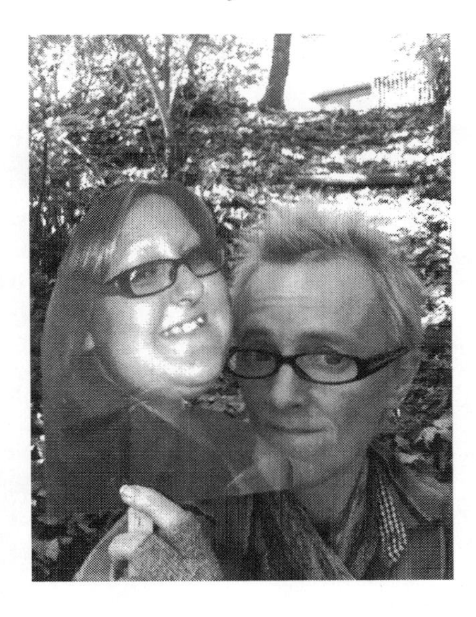

A Chemo Cocktail Chronology

2008

August 11 ..... Damn spot
August 12 ..... Dr. Allen
August 13 ..... Mammogram/ultrasound
August 14 ..... Breast thermography
August 15 ..... Dr. Stahl
August 19 ..... Lumpectomy/biopsy
August 20 ..... *C* word
August 23 ..... Prayer meeting/Dave's 43rd
August 26 ..... Pre-chemo 'do
August 28 ..... Youth group prayer meeting/bra burning
August 29 ..... Mastectomy
September 3 ..... Lymph node report: all clear
September 5 ..... Drainage tubes out
September 11 ..... First MUGA scan
September 12 ..... Stitches out
September 14 ..... Cincinnati Race for the Cure
September 16 ..... Bone/CT scan: all clear
September 17 ..... Genetic counseling: not genetic
September 25 ..... Port catheter surgery
September 27 ..... Praise meeting/Mm 43rd
September 29 ..... First chemo cocktail (Adriamycin/Cytoxin mix)
October 14 ..... Matt's sweet 16
October 15 ..... Oh where is my hairbrush?
November 10 ..... Last Adriamycin/Cytoxin chemo cocktail
November 24 ..... First Taxol chemo cocktail
November 28 ..... The darkest night of my soul Linda Wimmers R.I.P.
December 6 ..... Tiffany Foundation event/award
December 8 ..... First Herceptin/Taxol chemo cocktail mix
December 26 ..... Our 21st anniversary

2009

January 20 ..... Amanda's 18th
January 21 ..... Redheads come to last Taxol chemo cocktail
February 9 ..... First Herceptin-only cocktail
February 18 ..... MUGA scan
February 21 ..... Gramcracker's funeral
March 24 to 29 ..... Amanda's spring break girls' getaway

April 29 to May 5 .... Rome
May 4.......... Vespa incident
May 6.......... Back to the chemo grind
May 22.......... Mikeyy's 15th
June 19 to 22.......... Amanda's *American Idol* audition in Chicago
July 2.......... Dr. Stahl no peas in the pod!
August 17 to 23 .... D.C., NYC trip
August 23 .... Dave's 44th
August 29 .... One-year cancerversary surprise party
September 14 .... Cincinnati Race for the Cure
September 27 .... My lucky 44th
September 28 .... Enter my chemo sister Shelly
October 9 .... MUGA scan
October 14 .... Matt's 17th
November 13.......... Mum's *C*-day
December 5.......... Tiffany Foundation event
December 8.......... Mum's lumpectomy
December 15.......... Singles play-offs
December 16.......... Doubles play-offs
December 21.......... Last chemo cocktail
December 23 to January 2 .... Christmas vacation
December 26.......... Our 22nd anniversary

2010

January 6 .... Port Rafa is undocked and sails away
January 8 .... Not a Chemo Cocktail party
January 20.......... Amanda's 19th
February 1 .... First quarterly "maintenance" visit to the oncologist
February 2 .... *Lost* finale
February 4 .... Last MUGA scan
February 9 .... Scans: FREEBIRD!
Mum begins first of 33 radiation treatments
March 24 to 30 .... Mt. Hermon Writer's Conference
April 28.......... Word Bums Writer's Group
May 15.......... Matt and Mikeyy graduate (and me too! [Read: retire!])
May 17.......... Started Writing *SHAKEN NOT STIRRED* full time
May 22.......... Mikeyy's 16th
April 30 .... Model in Karen Wellington
Memorial Foundation fashion show fundraiser
June 11 .... Rocinante rode off into the sunset
August 11 .... Two-Year Cancerversary Bookreading Bash
Fundraiser for Mikeyy's YWAM mission trip
August 23 .... Dave's 45th

September 1 .... Fly with Mikeyy to Paris then to drop him off at the YWAM base for discipleship/ filmmaking school in Herrnhut, Germany
September 4 to 11 .... Another Roman holiday (this time I got my Vespa bag)
September 25 .... Cincinnati Race for the Cure
September 27 .... Yay for more birthdays! I turned 45
October 14 .... Matt's 18th
October 15 to 18 .... To NYC for international premiere of The SCAR Project with my chemo sister Shelly
December 4 to 11 .... Dave and I finally took our Caribbean holiday to Cancun, thanks to the Karen Wellington Foundation for LIVING with Cancer
December 13 to 28 .... Matt sent Matt to Germany to spend Christmas with Mikeyy

2011

January .... Finished first draft of *SHAKEN NOT STIRRED*
January 20 .... Amanda's 20th
February 4 .... Charleston, S.C. bookreading
March 2 .... Filmed Rescue Video about my cancer story at Vineyard Cincinnati
March 5 .... Modeled in Karen Wellington fashion show
April 1 .... Mikeyy returns home from YWAM mission trip
April 10 to 22 .... Amanda goes on mission trip with Beaded Hope to South Africa
April 16 .... Indy Race for the Cure with my mum
April 21 .... First SCAR Project Cincinnati Exhibit Committee Meeting
May 1 .... Walked half marathon in Cincinnati's Flying Pig
May 7 .... Ran my first 5K (Atlanta Race for the Cure with Celina)
May 14 .... Columbus Race for the Cure with Team Kickin' It with Kristi
May 22 .... Mikeyy's 17th
August 20 .... Three-year cancerversary
August 23 .... Dave's 46th
September 2 .... Matt moves to UC with Amanda
September 8 to 12 .... Work on *Strange Brand of Happy* movie set with Mikeyy
September 21 .... First day of classes for University of Cincinnati; all three Redheads in college
September 24 .... Cincinnati Race for the Cure

September 27 46
September 29 to October 2 .... The SCAR Project Cincinnati Exhibit
October 14 .... Matt's 19th
November 2011 .... *SHAKEN NOT STIRRED… A CHEMO COCKTAIL* – the book!

The Chemo Cocktail Mix Soundtrack Credits

Part I
Shaken Not Stirred

1. "Born" by Karin Bergquist and Linford Detweiler. © 2005 Back Porch Productions. Performed by Over the Rhine on *Drunkard's Prayer.*

2. "When the Stars Go Blue" by Ryan Adams. © 2006 Curb Records. Performed by Tim McGraw on *Greatest Hits Vol 2.*

3. "Help Me Out God" by David Ghazarian and Myron T Hsu. © 2001 Inpop Records. Performed by Superchick on *Karaoke Superstars.*

4. "I'm Too Sexy" by Richard Fairbrass, Fred Fairbrass, and Rob Manzoli. © 1992 Tug Records. Performed by Right Said Fred on *Up.*

5. "Brick House" by William King. © 1977 Motown. Performed by Commodores on *Commodores.*

6. "I Don't Know Why" by Amy Grant and Wayne Kirkpatrick. © 2003 Grant Girls Music LLC % The Loving Co. Performed by Amy Grant on *Simple Things.*

7. "Mother and Child Reunion" by Paul Simon. © 1972 Columbia Records. Performed by Paul Simon on *Paul Simon.*

8. "Save You" by Pierre Bouvier, Chuck Comeau, Jeff Stinco, David Desrosiers, Sebastien Lefebrve, and Arnold Lanni. © Lyrics@Warner/ Chappell Music, Inc. © 2008 Lava/Atlantic. Performed by Simple Plan on *Simple Plan.*

9. "The Glory of It All" by David W. Crowder. © 2007 Sparrow Records. Performed by David Crowder Band on *Remedy.*

10. "Man! I Feel Like a Woman!" by Mutt Lange and Shania Twain. © 1999 Mercury Nashville. Performed by Shania Twain on *Come on Over.*

11. "Fix You" by Chris Martin, Jonny Buckland, Guy Berryman, and Will Champion. © 2005 Parlophone. Performed by Cold Play on *X & Y.*

12. "Be Ok" by Ingrid Michaelson. © 2008 Cabin 24. Performed by Ingrid Michaelson on *Ingrid Michaelson.*

13. "Drunkard's Prayer" by Karin Bergquist and Linford Detweiler. © 2005 Back Porch Records. Performed by Over the Rhine on *Drunkard's Prayer.*

14. "Honey I'm Home" by Mutt Lange and Shania Twain. © 1997 Mercury Nashville. Performed by Shania Twain on *Come on Over.*

15. "Waiting on the Sun" by Jason Wade, Aniell. © 2002 Reprise/Squint. Performed by Sixpence None the Richer on *Divine Discontent.*

16. "Burn and Shine" by Owen Thomas. © 2002 EMI/Sparrow Records. Performed by The Elms on *Truth Soul Rock & Roll.*

17. "I Run for Life" by Melissa Etheridge. © 2005 Island Records. Performed by Melissa Etheridge on *Greatest Hits Road Less Traveled.*

18. "Come Sail Away" by Dennis Deyoung. © 1977 A&M. Performed by Styx on *The Grand Illusion.*

19. "Better Days" by John Rzeznik. © 2005 Warner Bros. Performed by Goo Goo Dolls on *Let Love In.*

Part II
The Chemo Cocktail Mix

20. "Everyday Is a Winding Road" by Sheryl Crow, Jeff Trott, and B. MacLeod. © 1996 Warner/Chappell. Performed by Sheryl Crow on *Sheryl Crow.*

21. "The Hairbrush Song" by Mike Nawrocki and Phil Vischer. © 1995 Lyrick Studios Performed by Larry the Cucumber on *Are You My Neighbor?*

22. "You're So Vain" by Carly Simon. © 1972 Elektra. Performed by Carly Simon on *No Secrets.*

23. "Hit Me with Your Best Shot" by Eddie Schwartz. © 1980 Chrysalis. Performed by Pat Benatar on *Crimes of Passion.*

24. "Beauty From Pain" by Patricia Elaine Brock, Brandon Estelle, David Ghazarian, and Myron T Hsu. © 2005 Inpop Records. © 2006 Columbia Performed by Superchick on *Beauty From Pain.*

25. "Breathe" by Bono and The Edge. © 2009 Island. Performed by U2 on *No Line on the Horizon.*

26. "Chemo Limo" by Regina Spektor. © 2005 Sire/Rhino. Performed by Regina Spektor on *Soviet Kitsch.*

27. "One More Round" by Alyssa, Lauren, Mary Ann, Rebecca and Vincent Barlow. © 2007 Fervent/Spirit-Led. Performed by Barlow Girl on *How Can We Be Silent.*

28. "Sweet Dreams (Are Made of This)" by Annie Lennox and David A. Stewart. © 1983 RCA. Performed by Eurythmics on *Sweet Dreams (Are Made of This)*

29. "Wind in My Hair" by Joules Evans. © 2010 Jagged Doctrine. Performed by Kicked in Fence on *The Cheesin' Moon.*

30. "That's Amore" by lyricist Jack Brooks and composer Harry Warren. © 1953 Capitol. Performed by Dean Martin on *Dean Martin.*

31. "Backwards" by Marcel Francois Chagnon and Tony Carl Mullins. © 2006 Lyric Street. Performed by Rascal Flatts on *Me and My Gang.*

32. "I'm On a Roll" by Karen Michelle Berquist and Linford J. Detweiler. © 2007 Great Speckled Dog. Performed by Over the Rhine on *The Trumpet Child.*

33. "Lucky Star" by Madonna. © 1984 Sire/Warner Bros. and © 1990 Warner Bros. Performed by Madonna on *Madonna* and *Like a Virgin.*

34. "Whip It" by Gerald Casale and Mark Mothersbaugh. © 1980 Warner Bros. Performed by Devo on *Freedom of Choice.*

35. "Hey Jude" by Lennon/McCartney. © 1968 Apple. Performed by The Beatles on *Hey Jude.*

36. "This Is Country Music" by Brad Paisley and Chris Dubois. © 2011 Arista Nashville. Performed by Brad Paisley on *This Is Country Music.*

37. "Cancer Is a Bitch" lyrics by Amanda Evans and music by Matt Evans. © 2010 Jagged Doctrine. Performed by The Kicked in Fence on *The Cheesin' Moon.*

Part III
Hangover

38. "Beautiful Things" by Michael and Lisa Gungor. © 2010 EMI Christian Music Publishing. Performed by The Michael Gungor Band on *Beautiful Things.*

39. "This is Not the End" by Gungor. © 2011 Brash Music. Performed by Gungor on *Ghosts Upon the Earth.*

Not a Chemo Cocktail Recipe

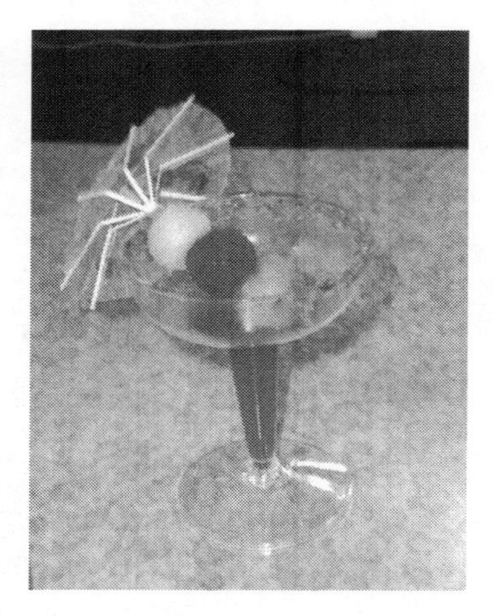

3 parts watermelon juice

1 part vodka

1 part melon liqueur (sweet or sour)

1 splash of cucumber juice

Shaken not stirred, of course

Umbrella skewer with watermelon, cantelope, and honeydew melon balls

Take a martini glass, lime the rim, dip it in Cosmopolitan rimmer

Let it pour and don't forget the umbrella

Cheers

In case you are one of those people who like to peek at the last page of the book I'll just cut to the chaser because it's 5 o'clock where I am, anyway. (For those of you who've already been there and back again with me through my cancer story you already knew that.) Regardless of how you got here, there's no judgment here, the point is: we're all here. So welcome, everyone, to the happy ending! I want you to know that I am lifting a glass, to you, and to your health.

I hope you're not having to toast with pink boxing gloves on. I know from experience how clumsy they can be when clinking cocktail glasses. I hope you picked up my book about cancer for some reason *other* than because you or someone you love has cancer. But if that's the case I'm praying for you right now while I type these words. I pray for healing. I pray that my words and the meditations of my heart contained in this book will be pleasing to God. And I pray that you may find some cheer here.

If you haven't worn pink boxing gloves I hope you never will, because let's face it, everybody is getting as sick and tired of pink as we all are of cancer.

Here's to a cure. Please, God, a cure.

And in the meantime, please go to second base and check yourself. This is not *meant* to be a cautionary tale. It *is* a comedy about my tragedy. It's my postcard from the other side of breast cancer and chemo: been there, done that, had to buy a new T-shirt. Don't wish you were here.

Here's to saving the ta-tas.

Made in the USA
Charleston, SC
23 April 2012